QM Medical Libraries

24 1015377 6

D0192098

BARTS AND THE LONDON

SCHOOL OF MEDICINE AND DENTISTRY

WHITECHAPEL LIBRARY,TURNER STREET, LONDON E1 2AD

020 7882 7110

ONE WEEK LOAN

Book are to be returned on or before the last date below,
otherwise fines may be charged.

3 0 MAR 2005

2 APR 2005

13 FEB 2006

3 1 JAN 2007

- 6 MAR 2006

2 7 FEB

- 9 DEC 2007

- 4 MAR 2008

water damaged as of
Feb 2007 (KL)

e to

s

A clinical guide to endodontics

Peter Carrotte
Clinical Lecturer, Department of Adult Dental Care,
Glasgow Dental Hospital and School,
378, Sauchiehall Street,
Glasgow G2 3JZ

Endodontic Specialist

2003
Published by the British Dental Association
64 Wimpole Street, London, W1G 8YS

Preface

Stock and Nehammer's *Endodontics in Practice* was first published in 1985, and almost immediately became a standard text for both undergraduate students and general practitioners. In the first sentence of the first chapter the authors observed '*during the last three decades research in the field of endodontics has modified the approach to treatment*', and that observation was retained in the extensively revised second edition, published in 1990.

With an inordinate amount of research of an increasingly high standard taking place, the changes in the field of endodontics during the last decade have been even greater. There are two consequences of this which relate to this textbook. The first is that a third edition is now required, to keep practitioners up to date with current thinking and practice. The second is that, because of their research commitments, Chris Stock and Carl Nehammer sadly do not have the time to devote to such a task.

I am therefore honoured and delighted to have edited this edition of their text. In some aspects of the subject there has been little change, whilst the developments in others have been immense. I may be criticized for retaining some historical material which could seem outdated to the modern practitioner using the latest canal preparation techniques. However, few dental schools have the resources necessary to introduce many of the recent developments, and undergraduate students still learn conventional techniques. It is important that they understand how these have developed, and it is essential, as with most things in life, that they develop basic skills before advanced ones!

The format of the book remains the same, indeed the preface to Stock and Nehammer's second edition, reproduced opposite, remains as valid today as it was then. This is a practical textbook written for the practice of endodontics. The research which underpins this practice is discussed where necessary, but the prime aim of the book is to guide practitioners through their everyday treatment of teeth with endodontic problems.

Preface to the second edition

This second edition of *Endodontics in Practice* has been extensively updated and expanded, in keeping with the needs of general practitioners and dental students for higher standards and information on more advanced techniques. The demands of patients are now directed far more frequently towards conserving teeth rather than extraction and prosthetic replacement, so that endodontics is becoming a part of the day-to-day routine. This requires the operator to have a far greater knowledge and expertise than was necessary only a few years ago. Re-root treatment, treating the elderly tooth, removing fractured instruments, mending perforations, and producing apical closure with calcium hydroxide, are techniques that every practitioner is expected to carry out. If the dentist does not have the necessary skills, patients will seek help elsewhere.

This book is designed to guide and instruct both the general practitioner and the dental undergraduate through the current techniques used in practice. Tedious research and lengthy explanations have been omitted in favour of the practical approach. After all, it is no good just talking about it to patients, you have to be able to do it.

Acknowledgements

This book would not have been written without the valuable assistance of my friend and colleague, Stephen Godfrey. Fifteen years ago he tutored me extensively in both postgraduate teaching and endodontics, and several of the images used as illustrations may originally have been his. In the course of an academic career one acquires pictures from a variety of sources, and in addition to Stephen I would particularly like to acknowledge Professor Richard Walker (who first fired my enthusiasm for endodontics) for Figure 1, Part 1; Dr Manar Elkhazindar for Figure 13, Part 12; and Professor Richard Welbury and Dr Marie-Therese Hosey for the figures and information used in Part 10. I must also thank Mr Neil Conduit, of QED Ltd., for his kind permission to reproduce the following figures from his company literature: Part 5, 2, 12, 17, 27, 28, 29; Part 6, 4; Part 7, 9; Part 8, 10 and Mr Grant Taylor for the line drawings.

Peter Carrotte
November 2003

Contents

SBRLSMD

CLASS MARK	WU230 CAR
CIRC TYPE	I WK
SUPPLIER	DAW 10/1/05 £35.45
READING LIST	
OLD ED CHECK	

© British Dental Journal 2003

All rights reserved. No part of this publication may be
reproduced, stored in a retrieval system, or transmitted in
any form or by any means electronic, mechanical,
photocopying, recording or otherwise, without either the
permission of the publishers or a licence permitting
restricted copying in the United Kingdom issued by the
Copyright Licensing Agency Ltd, 90 Tottenham Court
Road, London W1P 9HE

ISBN 0 904588 77 7 Softback
ISBN 0 904588 83 1 Hardback

Printed and bound by
Dennis Barber Limited, Lowestoft, Suffolk

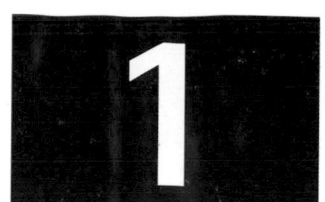
IN BRIEF

- Root canal treatment is normally prescribed to treat an infection, and as with all surgical procedures an aseptic technique is essential throughout.
- As research has shown that success is only achieved when all microorganisms are removed from the entire root canal system, the anatomy of this system must be understood for each tooth.
- Modern endodontic practice is concerned not with the old cliché of *cleaning, shaping* and *filling*, but with *shaping* first, to open the canals wide, so that *cleaning* can be effectively carried out prior to three-dimensional *filling*.

The modern concept of root canal treatment

Root canal treatment has changed considerably since the hollow tube theory was first postulated in 1930. Research continues into the elaborate anatomy of root canal systems, and also into the microbial causes of endodontically related diseases. Only by understanding these aspects in detail can the practitioner quickly and effectively *shape* the main root canals to facilitate thorough *cleaning* of the entire system, and easy and effective *filling*.

In 1965 Kakehashi, Stanley and Fitzgerald[1] showed conclusively that pulpal and endodontic problems are primarily related to microbial contamination of the root canal system. Since that time endodontology has increasingly focussed on the ways and means of eliminating microorganisms from the entire root canal system.

The majority of patients who require root canal treatment will have been diagnosed as suffering from the disease of periradicular periodontitis. The treatment of this disease must address the microbial contamination of the entire root canal system. It must also be carried out under aseptic conditions in order to prevent further microbial ingress, in particular from saliva. The use of a rubber dam very much reflects the use of a surgical drape in other invasive medical procedures. Such a biological approach will be emphasized throughout this text. The temptation to regard root canal treatment as a purely mechanical procedure, producing excellent post-operative radiographs but with little regard to diagnosis and prognosis, must be resisted in today's practice.

Research into the morphology of the pulp has shown the wide variety of shapes, and the occurrence of two or even three canals in a single root.[2] There is a high incidence of fins which run longitudinally within the wall of the canal and a network of communications between canals lying within the same root (Fig. 1). The many nooks and crannies within the root canal system make it impossible for any known technique, either chemical or mechanical, to render it totally sterile. The objective of treatment must be to reduce the level of microbial contamination as far as is practical, and to entomb any remaining microorganisms with an effective three-dimensional seal.

The prime aim when preparing the root canal has long been stated as *cleaning and shaping*. One of the prime aims of this text will be to encourage the practitioner to see this in reverse, ie *shaping and cleaning*. Modern instruments and techniques will be described which rapidly open and shape the main root

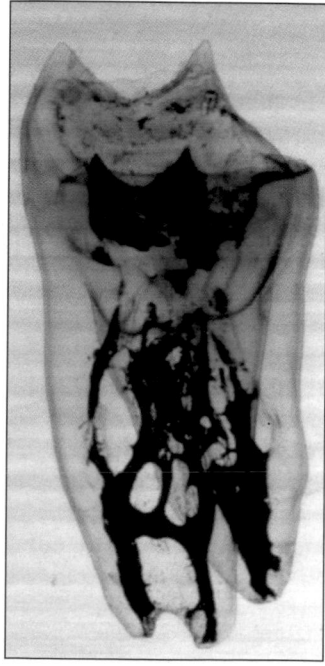

Fig. 1 The root canal system of this lower molar has been stained and the tooth totally decalcified, showing the complex nature of the root canal system. (Courtesy of Professor R T Walker.)

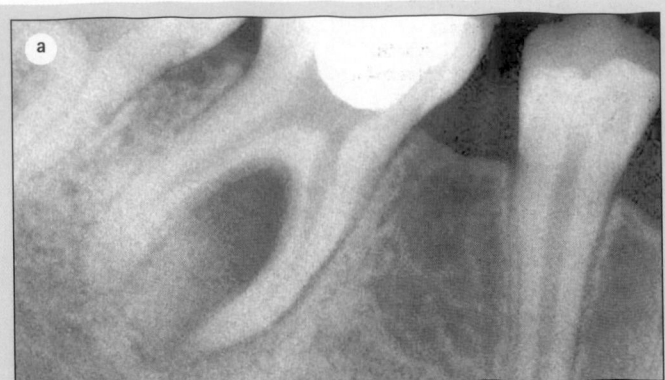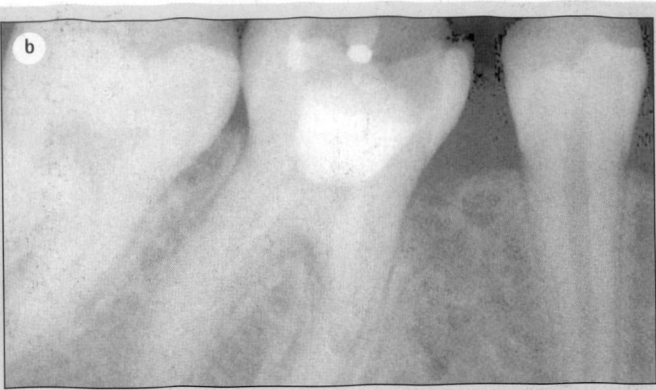

Fig. 2 (a) The pre-operative radiograph of tooth LR6 (46) shows a large radiolucent area associated with the root apex and the furcation area. Root canal treatment was commenced. (b) A radiograph 6 months later when the patient finally returned to continue treatment shows evidence of bony repair with a return to a normal periodontal ligament space around the apex and in the furcation.

canals, thus permitting the effective access of antimicrobial irrigants to the entire root canal system, including lateral canals, fins, anastamoses and other canal aberrations. It is imperative that these instruments are not seen as providing a route to quick and speedy root canal treatment. To achieve success the time saved by the rapid opening of the canal system must be spent in thorough and effective antimicrobial irrigation.

Research has also shown that when an infected root canal is accessed, the number of different species of microorganisms is small, rarely above single figures.[3] Treatment will become far more difficult and extended, and success may well be compromised, if this flora is altered by the ingress of saliva. Isolation of the tooth under treatment is essential not only for medicolegal reasons to protect the airway, but, far more importantly, to prevent further contamination of the root canal system and to permit the use of strong intracanal medicaments.

Other areas of research have had the significant effect of changing the approach to endodontic treatment. The hollow tube theory put forward by Rickert and Dixon in 1931[4] postulated that tissue fluids entering the root canal stagnated and formed toxic breakdown products which then passed out into the periapical tissues. This theory, that dead spaces within the body must be obturated, originally formed the basis for filling root canals. However, a variety of different studies have demonstrated that, on the contrary, hollow tubes are tolerated by the body. As a result there are currently two indications for filling a root canal, once the canal system has been shaped and cleaned. Firstly, to prevent the entry of microorganisms to the root canal system from either the oral cavity, should the coronal restoration leak or fail, or via the bloodstream (anachoresis). Secondly, to prevent the ingress of tissue fluid which would provide a culture medium for any bacteria remaining within the tooth following treatment.

A report by Klevant and Eggink[5] is particularly relevant. They shaped and cleaned a number of root canals, but the experimental group were not obturated. They ensured that an effective, well-sealed, coronal restoration was placed. They found that healing occurred in every case. Figure 2 shows a lower molar with a large periradicular lesion. The root canal system was shaped and cleaned, and an intervisit dressing of calcium hydroxide placed. The patient did not return for further treatment for 6 months, when a radiograph revealed that complete healing had taken place.

Of course, this does not mean that obturation is unimportant. It is essential for the reasons described earlier. It does prove, however, the old cliché that it is what is removed from the canal that is important, not what is put in. Similarly, Ray and Trope[6] found that root-treated teeth with a poor obturation on radiograph but a good coronal restoration had a better prognosis than teeth with a good obturation but a poor restoration.

The majority of root canal sealers are soluble and their only function is to fill the minute spaces between the wall of the root canal and the root filling material. Their importance, judged by the number of products advertised in the dental press, has been over-emphasized. Despite much research, gutta-percha remains the root filling of choice, although it is recognized that a biologically inert, insoluble and injectable paste may be better suited for obturation of the root canal. Most of the new root canal filling techniques are concerned with methods of heating gutta-percha, making it softer and easier to adapt to the irregular shape of the canal wall. It must be emphasized, however, that, whatever the obturation system used, if the root canal system has not been adequately cleaned healing may not occur (Fig. 3).

Finally, lesions of endodontic origin which appear radiographically as areas of radiolucency around the apices or lateral aspects of the roots of teeth are, in the majority of cases, sterile.[7,8] The lesions are the result of toxins produced by microorganisms lying within the root canal system. This finding suggests that the removal of microorganisms from the root canal followed by root filling is the first treatment of choice, and

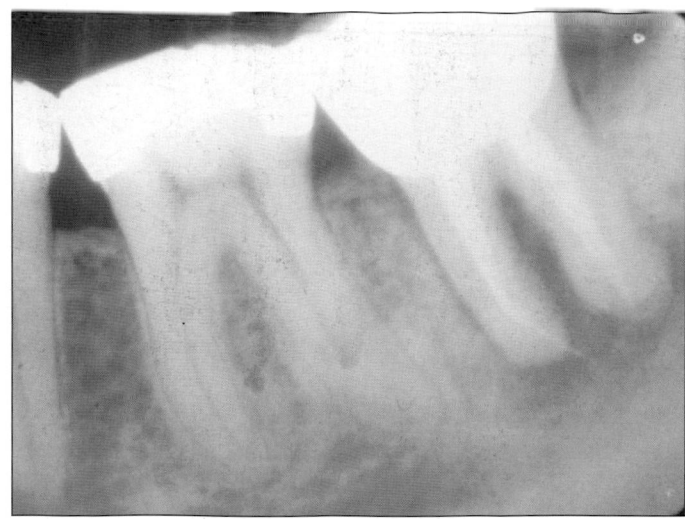

Fig 3 A radiograph of tooth LL7 (37) showing a root canal treatment carried out 12 months previously, with what appears to be an effective obturation yet no evidence of healing of the periradicular lesion.

that periradicular surgery, including an apicectomy with a retrograde filling, can only be second best.[9] Apicectomy with a retrograde filling at the apex is carried out in the hope of merely incarcerating microorganisms within the tooth, but does not take into account the fact that approximately 50% of teeth have at least one lateral canal. The long-term success rate of apicectomy must inevitably be lower than orthograde root treatment.

In summary, the principles of treatment of the disease of periapical periodontitis are as follows.

Shape: Produce a gradual smooth taper in the root canal with its widest part coronally and the narrowest part at the apical constriction, which, as discussed in Part 4, is normally about 1 mm short of the apex.

Clean: Use antimicrobial agents to remove microorganisms and pulpal debris from the entire root canal system.

Fill: Obturate the canal system with an inert, insoluble filling material.

1. Kakehashi S, Stanley H R, Fitzgerald R. The effects of surgical exposures of dental pulps in germfree and conventional laboratory rats. *J South California Dent Assoc* 1966; **334**: 449–451.
2. Burns R C, Herbranson E J. Tooth Morphology and Cavity Preparation, Chapter 7 in Cohen S and Burns R C, *Pathways of the Pulp*, St Louis 2002: Mosby.
3. Molven S, Olsen I, Kerekes K. Scanning electron microscopy of bacteria in endodontically treated teeth. III *In vivo* study. *J Endod* 1991; **7**: 226–229.
4. Rickert U G, Dixon C M. The controlling of root surgery. In *Transactions of the Eighth International Dental Congress*. Section 111a p15. Paris, 1931.
5. Klevant F J, Eggink C O. The effect of canal preparation on periapical disease. *Int Endod J* 1983; **16**: 68–75.
6. Ray H A, Trope M. Periapical status of endodontically treated teeth in relation to the technical quality of the root filling and the coronal restoration. *Int Endod J* 1995; **28**: 12–18.
7. Grossman L I. Bacteriologic status of periapical tissue in 150 cases of infected pulpless teeth. *J Endod* (Special Issue) 1982; **8**: 513–515.
8. Siqueira J F, Lopes H P. Bacteria on the apical root surfaces of untreated teeth with periradicular lesions: a scanning electron microscopy study. *Int Endod J* 2001; **34**: 216–220.
9. Pitt Ford T R. Surgical treatment of apical periodontitis. Chapter12 in Ørstavik D and Pitt Ford T R, *Essential Endodontology*. Oxford 1998: Blackwell.

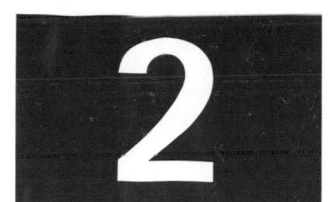

IN BRIEF

- An accurate diagnosis of the patient's condition is essential before an appropriate treatment plan can be formulated for that individual.
- A logical approach to clinical examination should be adopted.
- A high quality long-cone parallel radiograph is mandatory before commencing root canal treatment, and should be carefully examined to obtain all possible information.
- Root canal treatment may not be the most appropriate therapy, and treatment plans should take into account not only the expected prognosis but also the patient's dental condition, expectations and wishes.

Diagnosis and treatment planning

As with all dental treatment, a detailed treatment plan can only be drawn up when a correct and accurate diagnosis has been made. It is essential that a full medical, dental and demographic history be obtained, together with a thorough extra-oral and intra-oral examination. This part considers the classification of diseases of the dental pulp, together with various diagnostic aids to help in determining which condition is present, and the appropriate therapy.

The importance of correct diagnosis and treatment planning must not be underestimated. There are many causes of facial pain and the differential diagnosis can be both difficult and demanding. All the relevant information must be collected; this includes a case history and the results of both a clinical examination and diagnostic tests. The practitioner should be fully conversant with the prognosis for different endodontic clinical situations, discussed in Part 12. Only at this stage can the cause of the problem be determined, a diagnosis made, the appropriate treatments discussed with the patient and informed or valid consent obtained.

CASE HISTORY

The purpose of a case history is to discover whether the patient has any general or local condition that might alter the normal course of treatment. As with all courses of treatment, a comprehensive demographic, medical and previous dental history should be recorded. In addition, a description of the patient's symptoms in his or her own words and a history of relevant dental treatment should be noted.

Medical history

There are no medical conditions which specifically contra-indicate endodontic treatment, but there are several which require special care. The most relevant conditions are allergies, bleeding tendencies, cardiac disease, immune defects or patients taking drugs acting on the endocrine or CNS system. If there is any doubt about the state of health of a patient, his/her general medical

practitioner should be consulted before any endodontic treatment is commenced. This also applies if the patient is on medication, such as corticosteroids or an anticoagulant. An example of the particulars required on a patient's folder is illustrated in Table 1.

Antibiotic cover has been recommended for certain medical conditions, depending upon the complexity of the procedure and the degree of bacteraemia expected, but the type of antibiotic and the dosage are under continual review and dental practitioners should be aware of current opinion. The latest available edition of the *Dental Practitioners' Formulary*[1] should be consulted for the current recommended antibiotic regime. However, when treating patients whom may be considered predisposed to endocarditis, it may be advisable to liaise with the patient's cardiac

Table 1 A simple check list for a medical history (Scully and Cawson[2])

Anaemia
Bleeding disorders
Cardiorespiratory disorders
Drug treatment and allergies
Endocrine disease
Fits and faints
Gastrointestinal disorders
Hospital admissions and attendances
Infections
Jaundice or liver disease
Kidney disease
Likelihood of pregnancy or pregnancy itself

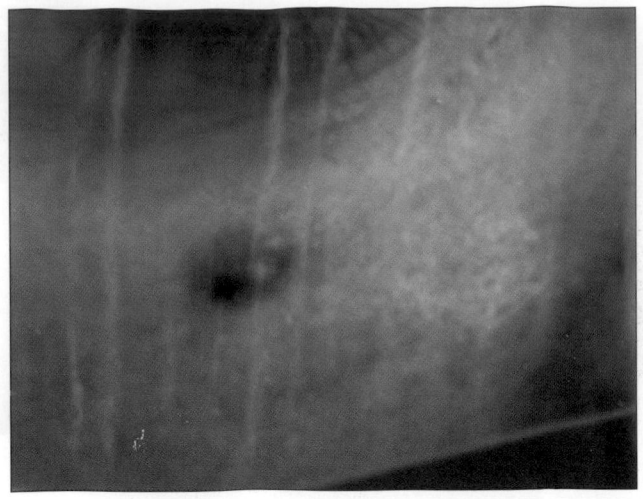

Fig. 1 A facial sinus associated with a severe periapical abscess on the upper canine.

specialist or general medical practitioner. Not all patients with cardiac lesions require antibiotic prophylaxis, and such regimes are not generally supported by the literature.[2] However, if it is agreed that the patient is at risk, they would normally be prescribed the appropriate prophylactic antibiotic regime, and should be advised to report even a minor febrile illness which occurs up to 2 months following root canal treatment. Prior to endodontic surgery, it is useful to prescribe aqueous chlorhexidine (2%) mouthwash.

Patient's complaints

Listening carefully to the patient's description of his/her symptoms can provide invaluable information. It is quicker and more efficient to ask patients specific, but not leading, questions about their pain. Examples of the type of questions which may be asked are given below.

1. How long have you had the pain?
2. Do you know which tooth it is?
3. What initiates the pain?
4. How would you describe the pain?
   Sharp or dull
   Throbbing
   Mild or severe
   Localized or radiating
5. How long does the pain last?
6. Does it hurt most during the day or night?
7. Does anything relieve the pain?

It is usually possible to decide, as a result of questioning the patient, whether the pain is of pulpal, periapical or periodontal origin, or if it is non-dental in origin. As it is not possible to diagnose the histological state of the pulp from the clinical signs and symptoms, the terms acute and chronic pulpitis are not appropriate. In cases of pulpitis, the decision the operator must make is whether the pulpal inflammation is reversible, in which case it may be treated conservatively, or irreversible, in which case either the pulp or the tooth must be removed, depending upon the patient's wishes.

If symptoms arise spontaneously, without stimulus, or continue for more than a few seconds after a stimulus is withdrawn, the pulp may be deemed to be irreversibly damaged. Applications of sedative dressings may relieve the pain, but the pulp will continue to die until root canal treatment becomes necessary. This may then prove more difficult if either the root canals have become infected or if sclerosis of the root canal system has occurred. The correct diagnosis, once made, must be adhered to with the appropriate treatment.

In early pulpitis the patient often cannot localize the pain to a particular tooth or jaw because the pulp does not contain any proprioceptive nerve endings. As the disease advances and the periapical region becomes involved, the tooth will become tender and the proprioceptive nerve endings in the periodontal ligament are stimulated.

CLINICAL EXAMINATION

A clinical examination of the patient is carried out after the case history has been completed. The temptation to start treatment on a tooth without examining the remaining dentition must be resisted. Problems must not be dealt with in isolation and any treatment plan should take the entire mouth and the patient's general medical condition and attitude into consideration.

Extra-oral examination

The patient's face and neck are examined and any swelling, tender areas, lymphadenopathy, or extra-oral sinuses noted, as shown in Figure 1.

Intra-oral examination

An assessment of the patient's general dental state is made, noting in particular the following aspects (Fig. 2).

- Standard of oral hygiene.
- Amount and quality of restorative work.
- Prevalence of caries.
- Missing and unopposed teeth.
- General periodontal condition.
- Presence of soft or hard swellings.
- Presence of any sinus tracts.
- Discoloured teeth.
- Tooth wear and facets.

Diagnostic tests

Most of the diagnostic tests used to assess the state of the pulp and periapical tissues are relatively crude and unreliable. No single test,

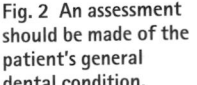

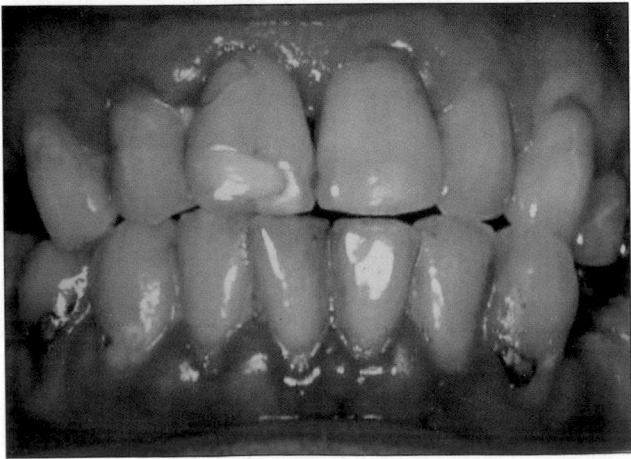

Fig. 2 An assessment should be made of the patient's general dental condition.

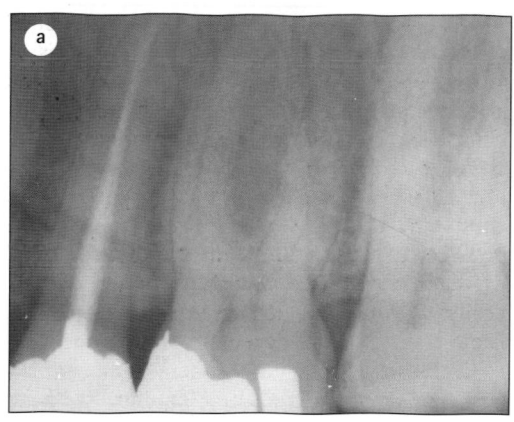

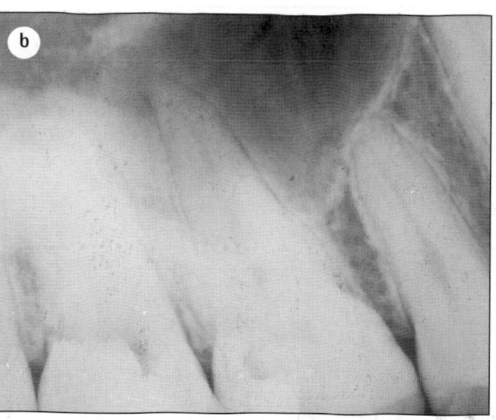

Fig. 3 The anatomical detail obtained from a radiograph taken by the long-cone paralleling technique (a) is far clearer and more accurate than when the bisecting angle technique (b) is used.

however positive the result, is sufficient to make a firm diagnosis of reversible or irreversible pulpitis. There is a general rule that before drilling into a pulp chamber there should be two independent positive diagnostic tests. An example would be a tooth not responding to the electric pulp tester and tender to percussion.

Palpation

The tissues overlying the apices of any suspect teeth are palpated to locate tender areas. The site and size of any soft or hard swellings are noted and examined for fluctuation and crepitus.

Percussion

Gentle tapping with a finger both laterally and vertically on a tooth is sufficient to elicit any tenderness. It is not necessary to strike the tooth with a mirror handle, as this invites a false-positive reaction from the patient.

Mobility

The mobility of a tooth is tested by placing a finger on either side of the crown and pushing with one finger while assessing any movement with the other. Mobility may be graded as:

1 – slight (normal)
2 – moderate
3 – extensive movement in a lateral or mesiodistal direction combined with a vertical displacement in the alveolus.

Radiography

In all endodontic cases, a good intra-oral parallel radiograph of the root and periapical region is mandatory. Radiography is the most reliable of all the diagnostic tests and provides the most valuable information. However, it must be emphasized that a poor quality radiograph not only fails to yield diagnostic information, but also, and more seriously, causes unnecessary radiation of the patient. The use of film holders, recommended by the National Radiographic Guidelines[3] and illustrated in Part 4, has two distinct advantages. Firstly a true image of the tooth, its length and anatomical features, is obtained (Fig. 3), and, secondly, subsequent films taken with the same holder can be more accurately compared, particularly at subsequent review when assessing the degree of healing of a periradicular lesion.

A radiograph may be the first indication of the presence of pathology (Fig. 4). A disadvantage of the use of radiography in diagnosis, however, can be that the early stages of pulpitis are not normally evident on the radiograph.

If a sinus is present and patent, a small-sized (about #40) gutta-percha point should be inserted and threaded, by rolling gently between the fingers, as far along the sinus tract as possible. If a radiograph is taken with the gutta-percha point in place, it will lead to an area of bone loss showing the cause of the problem (Fig. 5).

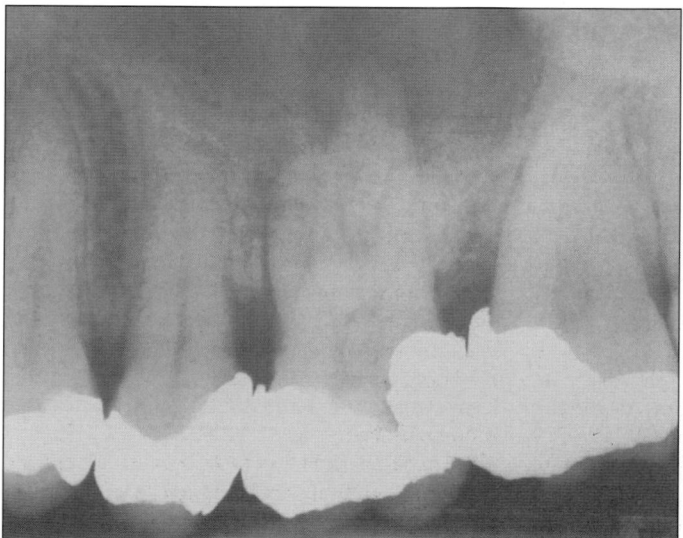

Fig. 4 A radiograph taken as part of a periodontal assessment also reveals a previously undiagnosed and asymptomatic periradicular lesion on the palatal root of tooth UL6 (26).

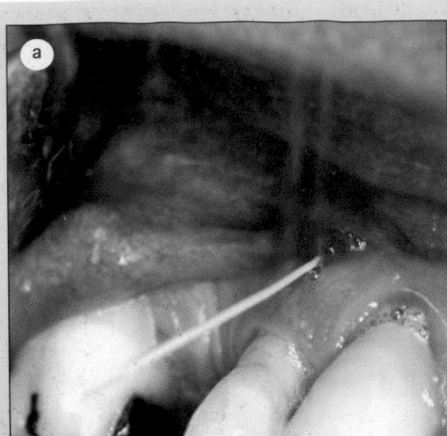

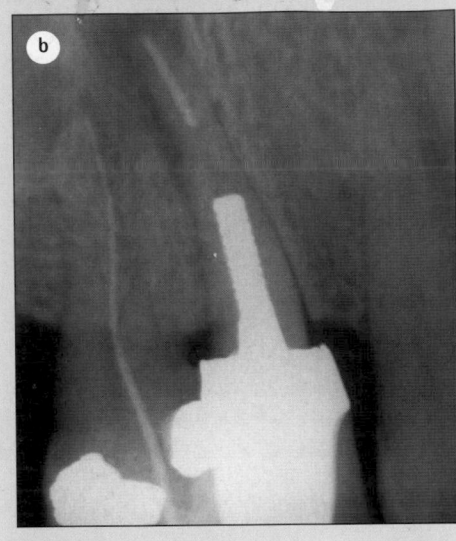

Fig. 5 A gutta-percha point has been threaded into a sinus tract adjacent to a recently root-treated canine (a). The radiograph (b) reveals the source of the infection to be the first premolar.

Pulp testing

Pulp testing is often referred to as 'vitality' testing. In fact, a moribund pulp may still give a positive reaction to one of the following tests as the nervous tissue may still function in extreme states of disease. It is also, of course, possible in a multirooted tooth for one root canal to be diseased, but another still capable of giving a vital response. Pulp testers should only be used to assess vital or non-vital pulps; they do not quantify disease, nor do they measure health and should not be used to judge the degree of pulpal disease. Pulp testing gives no indication of the state of the vascular supply which would more accurately indicate the degree of pulp vitality. The only way pulpal blood-flow may be measured is by using a Laser-Doppler Flow Meter, not usually available in general practice!

Doubt has been cast on the efficacy of pulp testing the corresponding tooth on the other side of the mid-line for comparison, and it is suggested that only the suspect teeth are tested.

Electronic The electric pulp tester is an instrument which uses gradations of electric current to excite a response from the nervous tissue within the pulp. Both alternating and direct current pulp testers are available, although there is little difference between them.

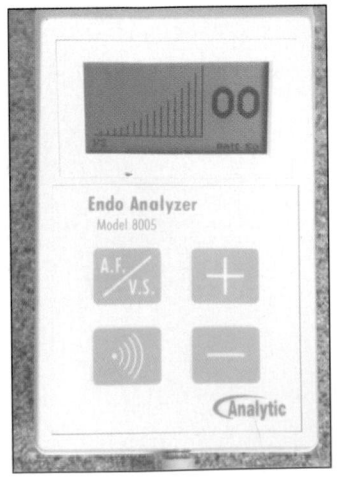

Fig. 6 A modern electric pulp tester combined with an endodontic apex locator.

Most pulp testers manufactured today are monopolar (Fig. 6).

As well as the concerns expressed earlier about pulp testing, electric pulp testers may give a false-positive reading due to stimulation of nerve fibres in the periodontium. Again, posterior teeth may give misleading readings since a combination of vital and non-vital root canal pulps may be present. The use of gloves in the treatment of all dental patients has produced problems with electric pulp testing. A lip electrode attachment is available which may be used, but a far simpler method is to ask the patient to hold on to the metal handle of the pulp tester. The patient is asked to let go of the handle if they feel a sensation in the tooth being tested.

The teeth to be tested are dried and isolated with cotton wool rolls. A conducting medium should be used; the one most readily available is toothpaste. Pulp testers should not be used on patients with pacemakers because of the possibility of electrical interference.

Teeth with full crowns present problems with pulp testing. A pulp tester is available with a special point fitting which may be placed between the crown and the gingival margin. There is little to commend the technique of cutting a window in the crown in order to pulp test.

Thermal pulp testing This involves applying either heat or cold to a tooth, but neither test is particularly reliable and may produce either false-positive or false-negative results.

Heat

There are several different methods of applying heat to a tooth. The tip of a gutta-percha stick may be heated in a flame and applied to a tooth. Take great note that hot gutta-percha may stick fast to enamel, and it is essential to coat the tooth with vaseline to prevent the gutta-percha sticking and causing unnecessary pain to the patient. Another method is to ask the patient to hold warm water in the mouth, which will act on all the teeth in the arch, or to isolate individual teeth with rubber dam and apply warm water directly to the suspected tooth. This is explored further under local anaesthesia.

Cold

Three different methods may be used to apply a cold stimulus to a tooth. The most effective is the use of a –50°C spray, which may be applied using a cotton pledget (Fig. 7). Alternatively, though less effectively, an ethyl chloride spray may be used. Finally, ice sticks may be made by filling the plastic covers from a hypodermic needle with water and placing in the freezing compartment of a refrigerator. When required for use one cover is warmed and removed to provide the ice stick. However, false readings may be obtained if the ice melts and flows onto the adjacent tissues.

Local anaesthetic

In cases where the patient cannot locate the pain and routine thermal tests have been negative, a reaction may be obtained by asking the patient to sip hot water from a cup. The patient is instructed to hold the water first against the mandibular teeth on one side and then by tilting the head, to include the maxillary teeth. If a reaction occurs, an intraligamental injection may be given to anaesthetise the suspect tooth and hot water is then again applied to the area; if there is no reaction, the pulpitic tooth has been identified. It should be borne in mind that a better term for intraligamental is intra-osseous, as the local anaesthetic will pass into the medullary spaces round the tooth and may possibly also affect the proximal teeth.

Wooden stick

If a patient complains of pain on chewing and there is no evidence of periapical inflammation, an incomplete fracture of the tooth may be suspected. Biting on a wood stick in these cases can elicit pain, usually on release of biting pressure.

Fibre-optic light

A powerful light can be used for transilluminating teeth to show interproximal caries, fracture, opacity or discoloration. To carry out the test, the dental light should be turned off and the fibre-optic light placed against the tooth at the gingival margin with the beam directed through the tooth. If the crown of the tooth is fractured, the light will pass through the tooth until it strikes the stain lying in the fracture line; the tooth beyond the fracture will appear darker.

Cutting a test cavity

When other tests have given an indeterminate result, a test cavity may be cut in a tooth which is believed to be pulpless. In the author's opinion, this test can be unreliable as the patient may give a positive response although the pulp is necrotic. This is because nerve tissues can continue to conduct impulses for some time in the absence of a blood supply.

TREATMENT PLANNING

Having taken the case history and carried out the relevant diagnostic tests, the patient's treatment is then planned. The type of endodontic treatment chosen must take into account the patient's medical condition and general dental state. The indications and contra-indications for root canal treatment are given below and the problems of re-root treatment discussed. The treatment of fractured instruments, perforations and perio-endo lesions are discussed in subsequent chapters.

It should be emphasized here that there is a considerable difference between *a treatment plan* and *planning treatment*. Figure 8 shows a radiograph of a patient with a severe endodontic problem. A diagnosis of failed root canal treatments, periapical periodontitis (both apically and also associated with a perforation of one root), and failed post crowns could be made. A *treatment plan* for this patient may be orthograde re-root canal treatment, with repair of the perforation, followed by the provision of new posts and cores, and crowns.

However, success in this case may depend upon the correct *planning of treatment*. For example, what provisional restorations will be used during the root canal treatment, and during the following re-evaluation period. Temporary post-crowns have been shown to be very poor at resisting microleakage.[4] The provision of a temporary over denture, enabling the total sealing of the access cavities, would seem an appropriate alternative, but if this has not been properly planned for, problems may arise and successful treatment may be compromised.

INDICATIONS FOR ROOT CANAL TREATMENT

All teeth with pulpal or periapical pathology are candidates for root canal treatment. There are also situations where elective root canal treatment is the treatment of choice.

Post space

A vital tooth may have insufficient tooth substance to retain a jacket crown so the tooth may have to be root-treated and restored with a post-retained crown (Fig. 9).

·Overdenture

Decoronated teeth retained in the arch to preserve alveolar bone and provide support or removable prostheses must be root-treated.

Teeth with doubtful pulps

Root treatment should be considered for any tooth with doubtful vitality if it requires an extensive restoration, particularly if it is to be a bridge abutment. Such elective root canal treatment has a good prognosis as the root canals are easy to access and are not infected. If the indications are ignored and the treatment deferred until the pulp becomes painful or even necrotic,

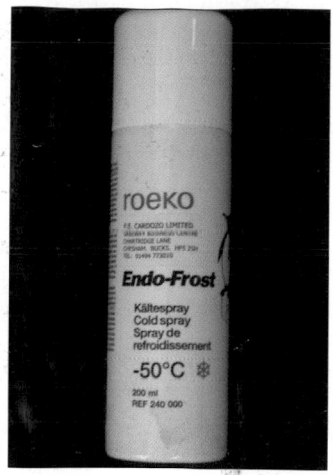

Fig. 7 A more effective source of cold stimulus for sensibility testing.

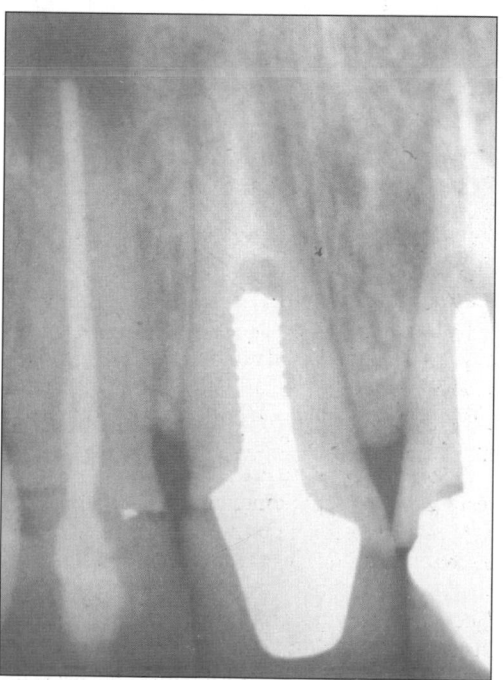

Fig. 8 This complicated case exhibits a number of different endodontic problems, and requires careful treatment planning if success is to be achieved.

Fig. 9 Tooth UL1 (21) requires a crown, but there is insufficient coronal tissue remaining. One possible treatment plan would be elective endodontic treatment followed by the provision of a post-retained core build-up and crown.

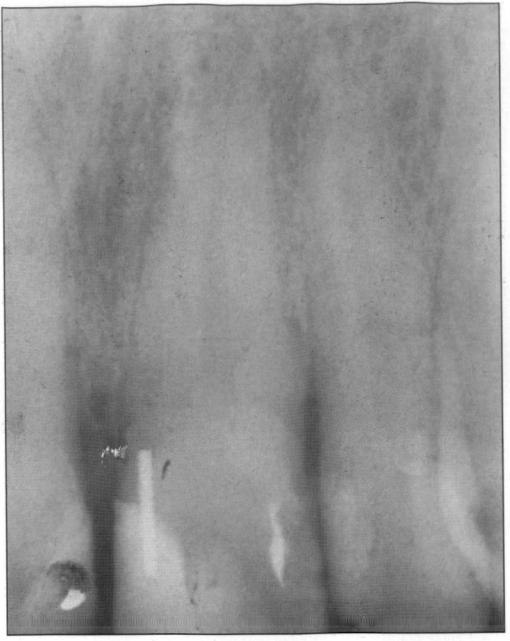

access through the crown or bridge will be more restricted, and treatment will be significantly more difficult, with a lower prognosis.[5]

Risk of exposure

Preparing teeth for crowning in order to align them in the dental arch can risk traumatic exposure. In some cases these teeth should be electively root-treated.

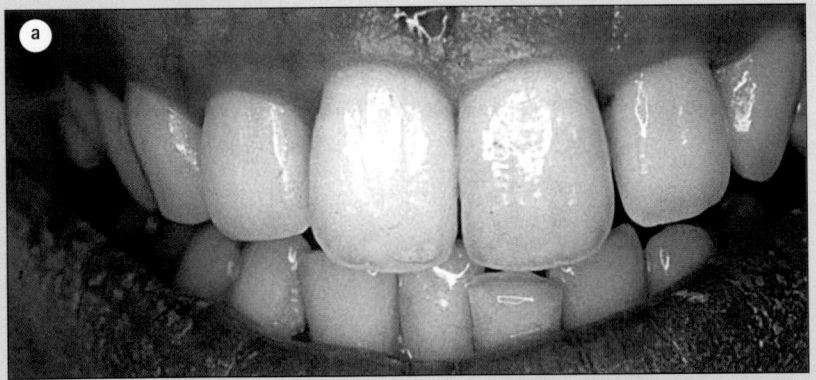

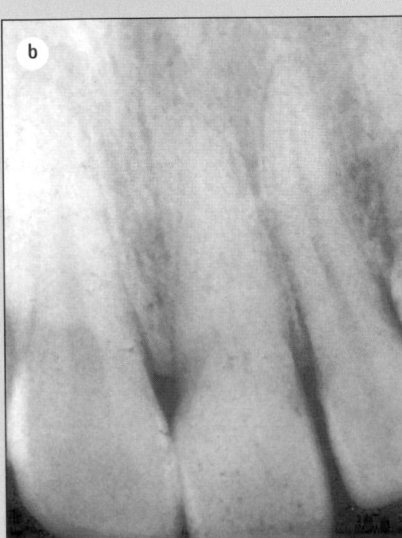

Fig. 10 A 23-year-old female patient suffered trauma to tooth UL1 (21) when aged 16, and is complaining about the yellow discoloration of the tooth (a). A radiograph (b) reveals that the pulp space has sclerosed.

Periodontal disease

In multirooted teeth there may be deep pocketing associated with one root or the furcation. The possibility of elective devitalization following the resection of a root should be considered (see Part 9).

Pulpal sclerosis following trauma

Review periapical radiographs should be taken of teeth which have been subject to trauma. If progressive narrowing of the pulp space is seen due to secondary dentine, elective root canal treatment may be considered while the coronal portion of the root canal is still patent. This may occasionally apply after a pulpotomy has been carried out. However, Andreasen[6] refers to a range of studies that show a maximum of 16% of sclerosed teeth subsequently cause problems, and the decision over root canal treatment must be arrived at after full consultation with the patient. If the sclerosing tooth is showing the classic associated discoloration the patient may elect for treatment, but otherwise the tooth may better be left alone (Fig. 10).

CONTRA-INDICATIONS TO ROOT CANAL TREATMENT

The medical conditions which require special precautions prior to root canal treatment have already been listed. There are, however, other conditions both general and local, which may contra-indicate root canal treatment.

General

Inadequate access

A patient with restricted opening or a small mouth may not allow sufficient access for root canal treatment. A rough guide is that it must be possible to place two fingers between the mandibular and maxillary incisor teeth so that there is good visual access to the areas to be treated. An assessment for posterior endodontic surgery may be made by retracting the cheek with a finger. If the operation site can be seen directly with ease, then the access is sufficient.

Poor oral hygiene

As a general rule root canal treatment should not be carried out unless the patient is able to maintain his/her mouth in a healthy state, or can be taught and motivated to do so. Exceptions may be patients who are medically or physically compromised, but any treatment afforded should always be in the best long-term interests of the patient.

Patient's general medical condition

The patient's physical or mental condition due to, for example, a chronic debilitating disease or old age, may preclude endodontic treatment. Similarly, the patient at high risk to infective endocarditis, for example one who has had a previous attack, may not be considered suitable for complex endodontic therapy.

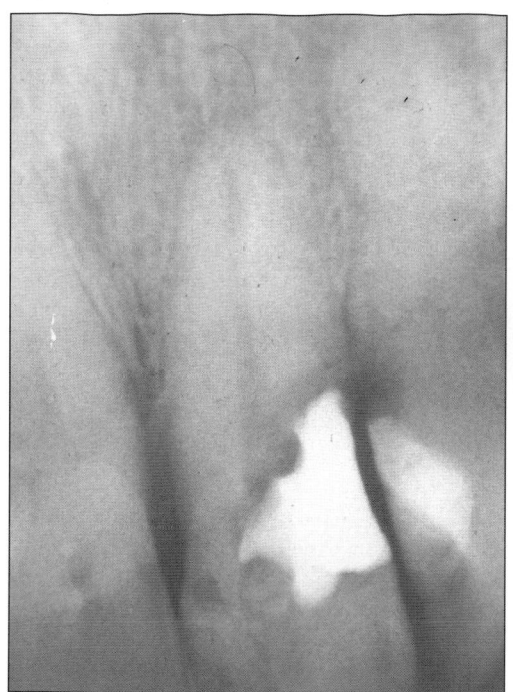

Fig. 11 Tooth UL1 (21) was so extensively decayed subgingivally that restoration would have proved impossible even if endodontic treatment had been carried out.

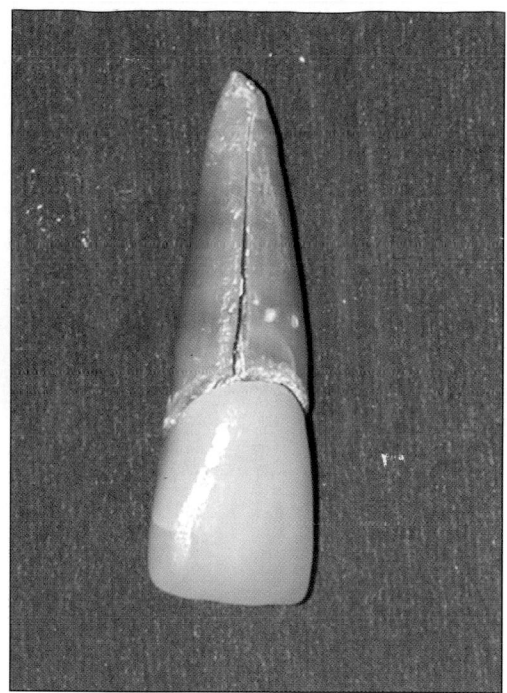

Fig. 12 The vertical root fracture can be clearly seen in this extracted tooth which had been fitted with a post crown.

Patient's attitude

Unless the patient is sufficiently well motivated, a simpler form of treatment is advised.

Local

Tooth not restorable

It must be possible, following root canal treatment, to restore the tooth to health and function (Fig. 11). The finishing line of the restoration must be supracrestal and preferably supragingival.

An assessment of possible restorative problems should always be made before root canal treatment is prescribed.

Insufficient periodontal support

Provided the tooth is functional and the attachment apparatus healthy, or can be made so, root canal treatment may be carried out.

Non-strategic tooth

Extraction should be considered rather than root canal treatment for unopposed and non-functional teeth.

Root fractures

Incomplete fractures of the root have a poor prognosis if the fracture line communicates with the oral cavity as it becomes infected. For this reason, vertical fractures will often require extraction of the tooth while horizontal root fractures have a more favourable prognosis (Fig. 12).

Internal or external resorption

Both types of resorption may eventually lead to pathological fracture of the tooth. Internal resorption ceases immediately the pulp is removed and, provided the tooth is sufficiently strong, it may be retained. Most forms of external resorption will continue (see Part 9) unless the defect can be repaired and made supragingival, or arrested with calcium hydroxide therapy.

Bizarre anatomy

Exceptionally curved roots (Fig. 13), dilacerated teeth, and congenital palatal grooves may all present considerable difficulties if root canal treatment is attempted. In addition, any unusual anatomical features related to the roots of the teeth should be noted as these may affect prognosis.

Re-root treatment

One problem which confronts the general dental practitioner is to decide whether an inadequate root treatment requires replacement (Fig. 14). The questions the operator should consider are given below.

1 Is there any evidence that the old root filling has failed?
   • Symptoms from the tooth.

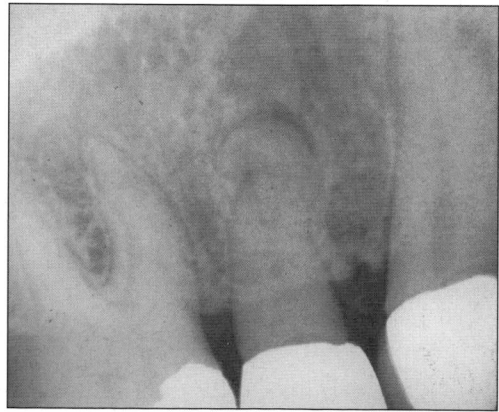

Fig. 13 The tooth UR4 (14) has such a bizarre root canal anatomy that endodontic treatment would probably be impossible.

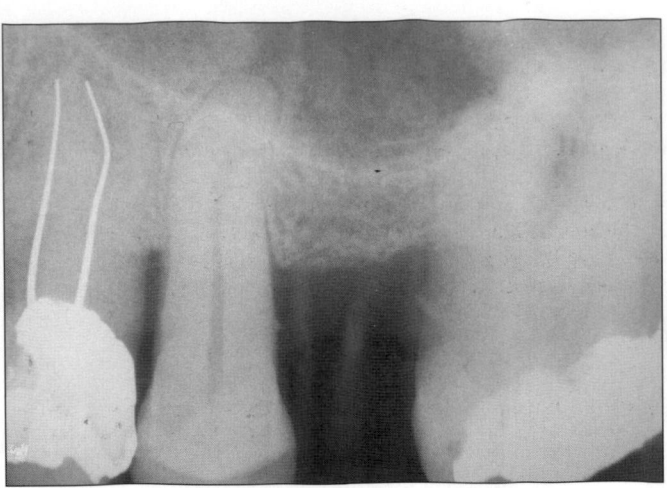

Fig. 14 Tooth UL4 (24) has previously been root treated (and obturated with silver points) but is symptomless. However, the tooth now requires a full crown restoration. A decision must be made as to whether the tooth should be re-treated before fitting the advanced restoration.

- Radiolucent area is still present or has increased in size.
- Presence of sinus tract.

2 Does the crown of the tooth need restoring?

3 Is there any obvious fault with the present root filling which could lead to failure?

Practitioners should be particularly aware of the prognosis of root canal re-treatments. As a rule of thumb, taking the average of the surveys reported in the endodontic literature (see Part 12) suggests a prognosis of 90–95% for an initial root canal treatment of a tooth with no radiographic evidence of a periradicular lesion. When such a lesion is present prognosis will fall to around 80–85%, and the longer the lesion has been present the more established will be the infection, treatment (ie removal of that infection from the entire root canal system) will be more difficult and the prognosis significantly lower. The average reported prognosis for re-treatment of a failed root canal filling of a tooth with a periradicular lesion falls to about 65%.

The final decision by the operator on the treatment plan for a patient should be governed by the level of his/her own skill and knowledge. General dental practitioners cannot become experts in all fields of dentistry and should learn to be aware of their own limitations. The treatment plan proposed should be one which the operator is confident he/she can carry out to a high standard.

1. *Dental Practitioners' Formulary* 2000/2002. British Dental Association. BMA Books, London
2. Scully C, Cawson R A. *Medical problems in dentistry.* Oxford: Butterworth-Heinemann, p74, 1998.
3. National Radiographic Protection Board. *Guidance Notes for Dental Practitioners on the safe use of x-ray equipment.* 2001. Department of Health, London, UK.
4. Fox K, Gutteridge D L. An *in vitro* study of coronal microleakage in root-canal-treated teeth restored by the post and core technique. *Int Endod J* 1997; 30: 361–368.
5. Ørstavik D. Time-course and risk analysis of the development and healing of chronic apical periodontitis in man. *Int Endod J* 1996; 29: 150–155.
6. Andreasen J O, Andreasen F M. Chapter 9 in *Textbook and colour atlas of traumatic injuries to the teeth.* 3rd Ed, Denmark, Munksgard 1994,.

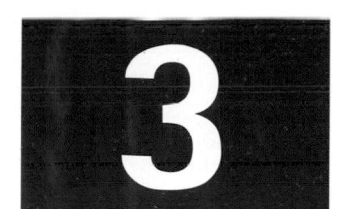

IN BRIEF

- Before any dental treatment is provided it is essential that the patient's symptoms have been correctly diagnosed.
- Conditions causing dental pain on first presentation may include pulpitis (reversible or irreversible), periapical periodontitis, dental abscess, as well as cracked tooth syndrome and other oro-facial pain disorders.
- Conditions arising during treatment may include high restorations, (probably the most common), root or crown fractures, problems with root canal instrumentation and infection.
- Following treatment pain may be due to any of the above, or failure of the root canal treatment. However, patients should always be cautioned to expect a certain amount of post-treatment discomfort.

Treatment of endodontic emergencies

The swift and correct diagnosis of emergency problems is essential when providing treatment, especially in a busy dental practice. A diagnosis must be made and appropriate treatment provided in usually just a few minutes. The sequence considered here encompasses problems presenting before, during and after dental treatment. Various diagnostic aids are considered, and some unusual presenting conditions discussed.

The aim of emergency endodontic treatment is to relieve pain and control any inflammation or infection that may be present. Although insufficient time may prevent ideal treatment from being carried out, the procedures followed should not prejudice any final treatment plan. It has been reported that nearly 90% of patients seeking emergency dental treatment have symptoms of pulpal or periapical disease.[1,2]

Patients who present as endodontic emergencies can be divided into three main groups.

Before treatment:

1. Pulpal pain
   a) Reversible pulpitis
   b) Irreversible pulpitis
2. Acute periapical abscess
3. Cracked tooth syndrome

Patients under treatment:

1. Recent restorative treatment
2. Periodontal treatment
3. Exposure of the pulp
4. Fracture of the root or crown
5. Pain as a result of instrumentation
   a) acute apical periodontitis
   b) Phoenix abscess

Post-endodontic treatment:

1. High restoration
2. Overfilling
3. Root filling
4. Root fracture

BEFORE TREATMENT

Details of the patient's complaint should be considered together with the medical history. The following points are particularly relevant and are covered more fully in Part 2.

1. Where is the pain?
2. When was the pain first noticed?
3. Description of the pain.
4. Under what circumstances does the pain occur?
5. Does anything relieve it?
6. Any associated tenderness or swelling.
7. Previous dental history:
   a) recent treatment;
   b) periodontal treatment;
   c) any history of trauma to the teeth.

Particular note should be made of any disorders which may affect the differential diagnosis of dental pain, such as myofascial pain dysfunction syndrome (MPD), neurological disorders such as trigeminal neuralgia, vascular pain syndromes and maxillary sinus disorders.

Diagnostic aids

- Periapical radiographs taken with a paralleling technique.
- Electric pulp tester for testing pulpal responses.
- Ice sticks, hot gutta-percha, cold spray and hot water for testing thermal responses.[3]
- Periodontal probe.

Pulpal pain

The histological state of the pulp cannot be assessed clinically.[4,5] Nevertheless, the signs and symptoms associated with progressive pulpal

Fig. 1 Initial radiographic assessment. Radiographs should be checked for any relevant information such as deep caries, pinned restorations, and the appearance of the periodontal ligament space.

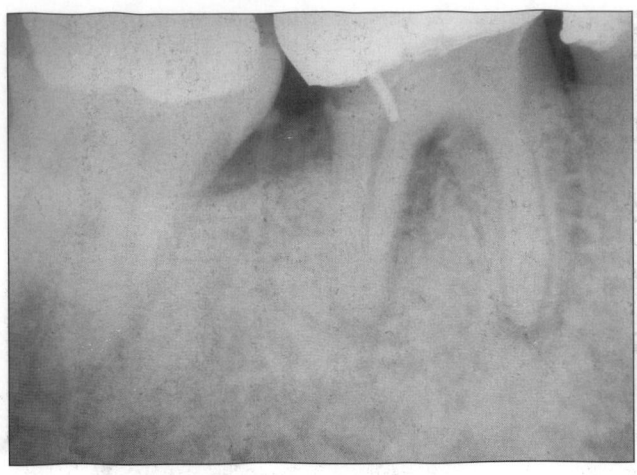

and periapical disease can give a reasonable indication of the likely state of an inflamed pulp, that is whether it is reversibly or irreversibly damaged.[6]

Irritation of the pulp causes inflammation, and the level of response will depend on the severity of the irritant. If it is mild, the inflammatory process may resolve in a similar fashion to that of other connective tissues; a layer of reparative dentine may be formed as protection from further injury. However, if the irritation is more severe, with extensive cellular destruction, further inflammatory changes involving the rest of the pulp will take place, which could eventually lead to total pulp necrosis.

There are features of pulpitis which can make the borderline between reversible and irreversible pulpitis difficult to determine clinically. In general, if the responses to several tests are exaggerated, then an irreversible state is possible.

The essential feature of a reversible pulpitis is that pain ceases as soon as the stimulus is removed, whether it is caused by hot or cold fluids, or sweet food. The teeth are not tender to percussion, except when occlusal trauma is a factor. Initially, one of the following treatment may be all that is necessary:

- Check the occlusion and remove non-working facets.
- Place a sedative dressing in a cavity after removal of deep caries.
- Apply a fluoride varnish or a dentine bonding resin to sensitive dentine and prescribe a desensitizing toothpaste.

Should the symptoms persist and the level of pain increase in duration and intensity, then the pulpitis is likely to be irreversible. The patient may be unable to decide which tooth is causing the problem, since the pain is often referred to teeth in both the upper and lower jaw on the same side. In the early stages, the tooth may exhibit a prolonged reaction to both hot and cold fluids, but is not necessarily tender to percussion. When testing for sensitivity to percussion it is not necessary to tap the tooth with the handle of dental instrument. Gentle finger pressure will be more than sufficient to elicit a response, and much kinder to your patient.

Only when the inflammation has spread throughout the pulp and has involved the periodontal ligament, will the tooth become tender to bite on. In these circumstances, the application of heat will cause prolonged pain which may be relieved by cold. Both hot and cold can precipitate a severe bout of pain, but as a rule heat tends to be more significant.

Pain from an irreversibly damaged pulp can be spontaneous and may last from a few seconds to several hours. A characteristic feature of an irreversible pulpitis is when a patient is woken at night by toothache. Even so, if untreated a symptomatic pulpitis may become symptomless and pulp tests may give equivocal results. In time, total pulp necrosis may ensue, without the development of further symptoms and the first indication of an irreversibly damaged pulp may be seen as a periapical rarefaction on a radiograph, or the patient may present with an acute periapical abscess.

To summarize, therefore, in reversible pulpitis:

- The pain is of very short duration and does not linger after the stimulus has been removed.
- The tooth is not tender to percussion.
- The pain may be difficult to localize.
- The tooth may give an exaggerated response to vitality tests.
- The radiographs present with a normal appearance, and there is no apparent widening of the periodontal ligaments.

In irreversible pulpitis:

- There is often a history of spontaneous bouts of pain which may last from a few seconds up to several hours.
- When hot or cold fluids are applied, the pain elicited will be prolonged. In the later stages, heat will be more significant; cold may relieve the pain.
- Pain may radiate initially, but once the periodontal ligament has become involved, the patient will be able to locate the tooth.
- The tooth becomes tender to percussion once inflammation has spread to the periodontal ligament.
- A widened periodontal ligament may be seen on the radiographs in the later stages.

Careful evaluation of a patient's dental history and of each test is important. Any one test on its own is an insufficient basis on which to make a diagnosis. Records and radiographs should first be checked for any relevant information such as deep caries, pinned restorations, and the appearance of the periodontal ligament space (Fig. 1). Vitality tests can be misleading, as various factors have to be taken into account. For example, the response in an older person may differ from that in someone younger due to secondary dentine deposition and other atrophic changes in the pulp tissue. Electric pulp testing is simply an indication of the presence of vital nerve tissue in the root canal system only and not an indication of the state of health of the pulp tissue.

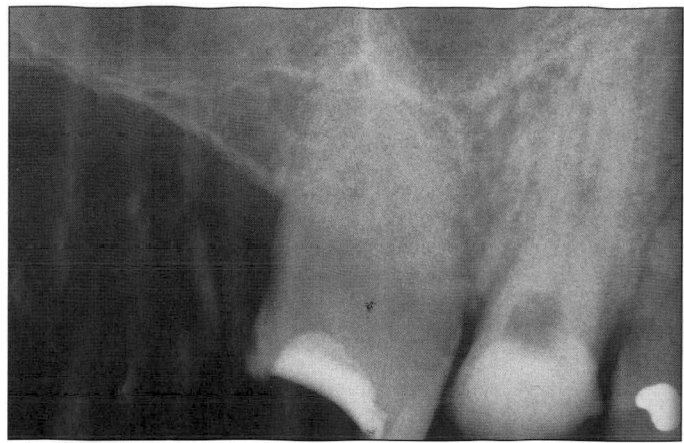

Fig. 2 Radiographic changes range from a widening of the periodontal ligament space (note that this upper first premolar has two separate buccal roots)...

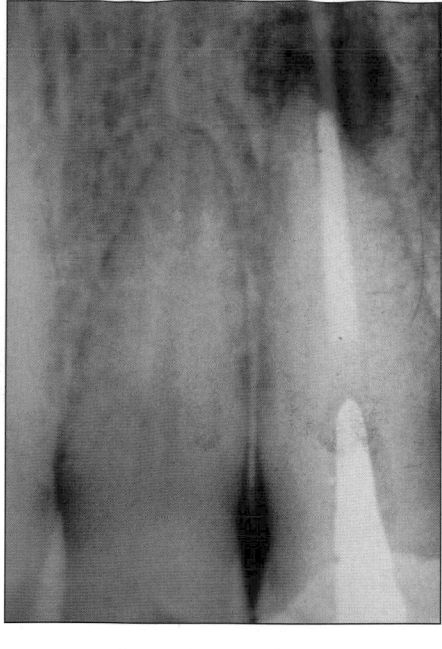

Fig. 3 ... to a large, well-defined area of radiolucency.

Once pulpal inflammation has spread to the periodontal ligament, the resulting inflammatory exudate may cause extrusion of the tooth, making it tender to bite on. This particular symptom, acute apical periodontitis, may be a consequence of occlusal trauma; the occlusion must therefore always be checked.

Ideally, the treatment for irreversible pulpitis is pulp extirpation followed by cleaning and preparation of the root canal system. If time does not permit this, then removal of pulp tissue from the pulp chamber and from the coronal part of the root canal is often effective. Irrigation of the pulp chamber using a solution of sodium hypochlorite before carrying out any instrumentation is important. (Sodium hypochlorite is usually sold as a 5% solution. This may be diluted with purified water BP to the operator's preference.) Sodium hypochlorite solution has proved to be one of the most effective disinfecting agents used in root canal treatment,[7,8] with different authors recommending strengths between 0.5 and 5.0%. The pulp chamber and root canals are dried, and a dry sterile cotton wool pledget placed in the pulp chamber with a temporary filling to seal the access cavity. Antiseptic solutions such as phenolic solutions or corticosteroid/ antibiotic preparations on cotton wool pledgets have been advocated, but their effectiveness is of doubtful value. Corticosteroid dressings should be used sparingly as there is evidence that suppression of an inflammatory response by steroids allows bacteria to enter the bloodstream with ease.[9] This is a particularly undesirable effect in patients who, for example, have a history of rheumatic fever. Studies have shown that provided the pulp chamber and the root canals have been cleansed and dried, medication of the pulp chamber and root canals is of little practical benefit. Paper points are used to dry the canals and under no circumstances should they be left in the canal, otherwise any fluid that enters the canal system will be absorbed and so provide an effective culture medium for any residual bacteria.

Difficulty with local analgesia is a common problem with an acutely inflamed pulp. In addition to standard techniques, supplementary analgesia can be obtained with the following:

1 Additional infiltration anaesthesia, such as long-buccal, lingual and palatal.
2 Intraligamental (intra-osseous) injection.
3 True intra-osseous injection.
4 Intrapulpal analgesia.
5 Inhalational sedation with local analgesia.

Should these techniques give only moderate success, it is advisable to dress the pulp to allow the inflammation to subside and to postpone pulp extirpation. A corticosteroid/antibiotic preparation with a zinc oxide/eugenol temporary restoration will provide an effective, short-term dressing.

Continuation of pain following pulp extirpation may be due to one of the following causes.

1 The temporary filling is high.
2 Infected pulp tissue is present in the canal.
3 Some of the canal contents have been extruded through the apex.
4 Overinstrumentation of the apex or perforation of the canal wall.
5 An extra canal may be present which has not been cleaned.

If the problem is not found to be occlusal, whatever the cause the remedy is to irrigate the pulp chamber and root canal system again with sodium hypochlorite solution and perhaps gently instrument, then dry and redress the tooth as before.

Acute periapical abscess

This condition develops from an acute periapical periodontitis. In the early stages, the difference between the two is not always clear. Radiographic changes range from a widening of the periodontal ligament space (Fig. 2), to a well-defined area (Fig. 3). The typical symptoms of an acute periapical abscess are a pronounced

Fig. 4 A pronounced
swelling may be
present adjacent to the
abscessed tooth.

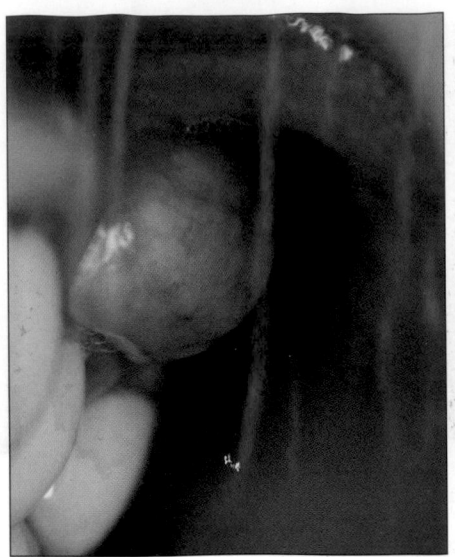

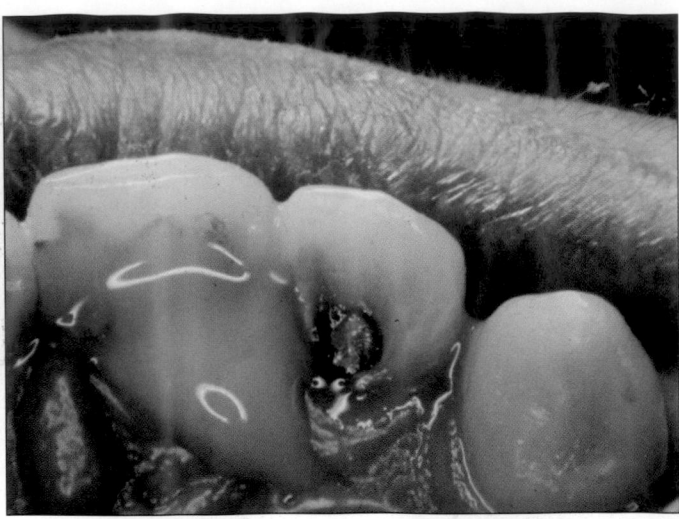

Fig. 5 Immediate relief is obtained as pus drains feely from an access cavity.

soft-tissue swelling (Fig. 4) and an exquisitely tender tooth. Extrusion from the socket will often cause the tooth to be mobile. Differential diagnosis of a suspected periapical swelling is important in case the cause is a lateral periodontal abscess. The diagnosis can be made by testing the vitality of the tooth. If it is vital, then the cause may well be periodontal in origin.

The immediate task is to relieve pressure by establishing drainage, and in the majority of cases this can be achieved by first opening up the pulp chamber, as seen in Figure 5. Initially, gaining access can be difficult because the tooth is often extremely tender. Gently grip the tooth and use a small, round, diamond bur in a turbine to reduce the trauma of the operation. Regional analgesia may be necessary, and inhalation sedation can prove invaluable. If drainage is not immediate it is permissible to explore the apical foramen with a very fine (size 08 or 10) file. The foramen should not be instrumented or enlarged, and if drainage does not result the procedure should not be persevered. As discussed in Part 7, the use of ultrasonically activated endodontic files may be particularly helpful in this situation for effectively flushing infected debris from the root canal system.

If a soft-tissue swelling is present and pointing intra-orally, then it may be incised to establish drainage as well. The presence of a cellulitis may result in little or no drainage. If a cellulitis is present, medical advice should be sought before any treatment is carried out (Fig. 6).

Incision to establish drainage

Incision to establish drainage is the only surgical endodontic procedure which may be undertaken when acute inflammation is present. The principal indication is the presence of a collection of pus which points from a fluctuant abscess in the soft tissues. Establishing drainage to help bring the infection under control is essential, and should always be obtained through the root canal and soft tissues in preference to administering antibiotics alone. The

soft-tissue swelling should be examined to see if it is fluctuant. Where the swelling is pointing intra-orally, copious amounts of surface analgesia should be applied, for example ethyl chloride or topical lignocaine ointment. Regional anaesthesia may not be effective due to the presence of pus, and the administration of a local analgesic solution may spread the infection further into the tissues.

Incise the swelling with a Bard–Parker No. 11 or 15 scalpel blade, or aspirate, using a wide-bore needle and disposable syringe. It may be possible to aspirate the abscess via the root canal as well. The advantage of this technique is that the sample can be sent for bacteriological examination if required. It is not usually necessary to insert a drain, but if it is thought necessary then a piece of quarter-inch or half-inch selvedge gauze may be used. The same criteria apply when extra-oral drainage is indicated, and it may be possible to use the same technique of aspiration with a wide-bore needle and disposable syringe. However, if an extra-oral incision is considered necessary, as in Figure 7, it is wise to refer the patient to an oral surgeon for this particular procedure.

Root canal treatment

Once access and initial drainage have been achieved, a rubber dam should be applied to the tooth to complete the operation. Before any further instrumentation is carried out, the pulp chamber should be thoroughly irrigated with a solution of sodium hypochlorite to remove as much superficial organic and inorganic debris as possible. This in itself may bring considerable pain relief and will make subsequent instrumentation easier. Having debrided the canals to the best possible extent with frequent changes of irrigant, the canals should be dried with paper points and a dry sterile cotton wool pledget placed in the pulp chamber to prevent ingress of the temporary dressing. The access cavity is then sealed to prevent re-infection of the canals from the oral cavity. If complete debridement was not possible the patient must

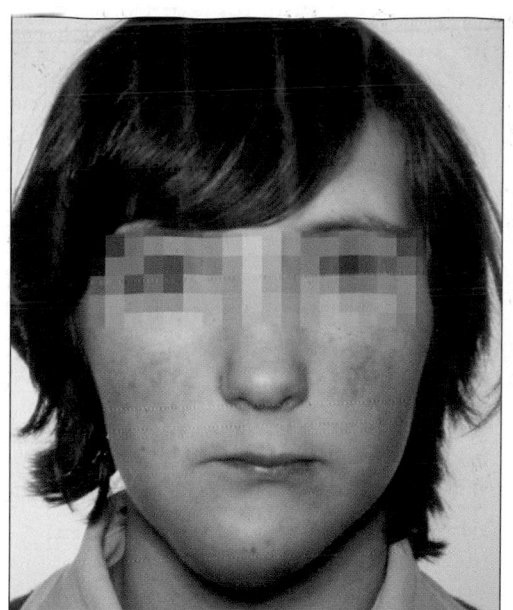

Fig. 6 A teenage patient who had a large periapical lesion of a lower incisor is developing a cellulitis.

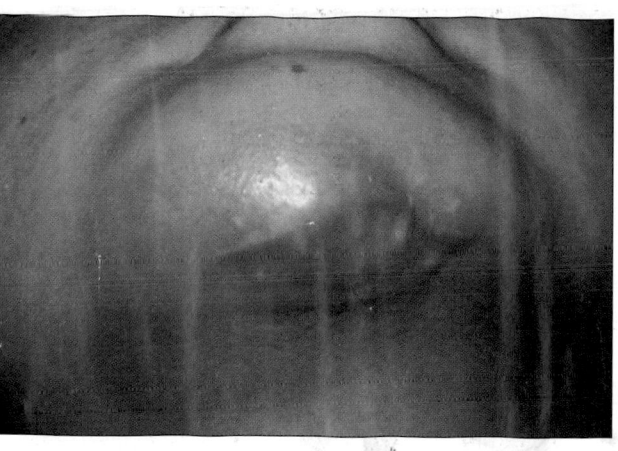

Fig. 7 External incision may be required, and the patient should preferably be referred to a general surgeon.

be recalled within 48 hours. At this time it will usually be possible to complete instrumentation and place a calcium hydroxide dressing in the canals.

The temptation to leave the tooth open to drain must be resisted at all costs.[10] The microbial flora of the canal will be changed, making treatment more difficult and lowering the long-term prognosis. Furthermore, this treatment contravenes the prime objective of treatment: to disinfect the root canal. If the clinician does not have sufficient time to carry out adequate treatment when opening the tooth, good clinical practice would suggest re-appointing the patient to the end of the treatment session when time is available.

Antibiotics are only required when there is systemic spread of the infection, the patient is unwell and has a raised temperature. Antibiotics are not an alternative to appropriate cleaning and disinfection of the root canal.[11] There is a serious tendency to over prescription of antibiotics in situations where they are not indicated. If, however, there is a clinical reason for their use, amoxycillin is usually the agent of choice, prescribing 250 mg three times a day until the infection is under control and root canal therapy initiated. Metronidazole is a useful alternative where the penicillins are contra-indicated.

CRACKED TOOTH SYNDROME (POSTERIOR TEETH)

Crazing of the enamel surface is a common finding on teeth as a consequence of function, but on occasion it may indicate a cracked tooth. If the crack runs deep into dentine and is therefore a fracture, chewing may be painful. Initially, this may not be of sufficient intensity for the patient to seek treatment. However, once the fracture line communicates with the pulp, pulpitis will ensue. A quiescent period of several months may

follow before any further symptoms develop. The patient may present with a whole range of bizarre symptoms, many of which are similar to those of irreversible pulpitis:

- Pain on chewing.
- Sensitivity to hot and cold fluids.
- Pain which is difficult to localize.
- Pain referred along to the areas served by the fifth cranial nerve.
- Acute pulpal pain.
- Alveolar abscess.

Diagnosis can be difficult and much depends on the plane of the fracture line and its site on the tooth. Radiographs are unlikely to reveal a fracture unless it runs in a buccolingual plane. A fibre-optic light is a useful aid as it will often reveal the position of the fracture. One diagnostic test is to ask the patient to bite on a piece of folded rubber dam. Care must be exercised as this test may extend the fracture line. The extent of the fracture line and its site will decide whether the tooth can be saved or not. If it is a vertical fracture, involves the root canal system and extends below the level of the alveolar crest, then the prognosis is poor and extraction is indicated (Fig. 8). However, if the fracture line is horizontal or diagonal and superficial to the alveolar crest, then the prognosis may be better.

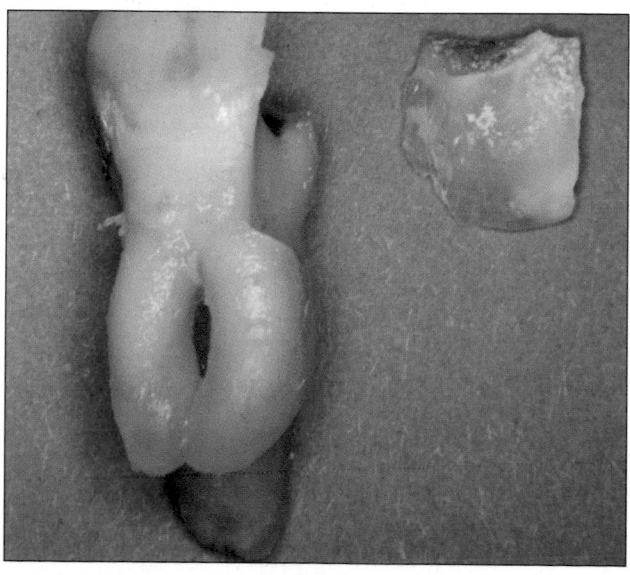

Fig 8 A patient who complained of classic 'cracked-cusp' pain was found to have such a deep subgingival cusp fracture that the tooth was extracted.

PATIENTS UNDER TREATMENT

Following endodontic procedures, patients may sometimes experience pain no matter how carefully the treatment has been given. It would be prudent to warn every patient to expect a certain amount of discomfort following endodontic treatment, advising them that this is caused by an inflammatory response at the tooth apex. They should be advised to take over-the-counter analgesics, preferably NSAIDs. However, if the pain persists for more than two or three days, further treatment is probably required for one of the following reasons.

Recent restorations

Pain may be a result of:

- High filling
- Microleakage
- Micro-exposure of the pulp
- Thermal or mechanical injury during cavity preparation or an inadequate lining under metallic restorations
- Chemical irritation from lining or filling materials
- Electrical effect of dissimilar metals.

It is not always possible to know beforehand whether there is a pre-existing pulpal condition when operative procedures are undertaken. Consequently, a chronic pulpitis may be converted into an acute pulpitis.

Periodontal treatment

There is always a chance that some of the numerous lateral canals that communicate with the periodontal ligament are exposed when periodontal treatment is carried out. This aspect is considered in the section in Part 9 on 'perio-endo lesions'.

Exposure of the pulp

If a carious exposure is suspected, then removal of deep caries should be carried out under rubber dam. The decision to extirpate the pulp or carry out either a pulp capping or partial pulpotomy procedure depends on whether the pulp has been irreversibly damaged or not (see Part 9 – calcium hydroxide). If there is insufficient time, or any difficulty is experienced with analgesia, temporary treatment, as recommended for irreversible pulpitis, may be carried out.

Root or crown fractures

Most root or crown fractures can be avoided by adequately protecting the tooth during a course of root canal treatment. If the structure of the tooth is damaged between appointments, pain is likely to occur as a result of salivary and bacterial contamination of the root canal. If the tooth happens to fracture in a vertical plane, the prognosis is poor and the tooth may have to be extracted (Fig. 9). In the case of multirooted teeth, it may be possible to section the tooth and remove one of the roots.

Pain as a result of instrumentation

The two conditions that may require emergency treatment during a course of root canal treatment are:

- acute apical periodontitis;
- Phoenix abscess.

Acute apical periodontitis may arise as a result of over instrumentation, extrusion of the canal contents through the apex, leaving the tooth in traumatic occlusion, or placing too much medicament in the pulp chamber as an inter-appointment dressing.

Irrigation of the canal with sodium hypochlorite and careful drying with paper points is usually sufficient to alleviate the symptoms. The occlusion must be checked, as there is likely to be a certain amount of extrusion of the tooth from its socket.

The term 'Phoenix abscess' relates to the sudden exacerbation of a previously symptomless periradicular lesion. It can be one of the most troublesome conditions to deal with and occurs after initial instrumentation of a tooth with a pre-existing chronic periapical lesion (Fig. 10). The reasons for this phenomenon are not fully understood, but it is thought to be due to an alteration of the internal environment of the root canal space during instrumentation which activates the bacterial flora. Research has shown that the bacteriology of necrotic root canals is more complex than was previously thought, in particular the role played by anaerobic organisms.

Treatment consists of irrigation, debridement of the root canal and establishing drainage. In

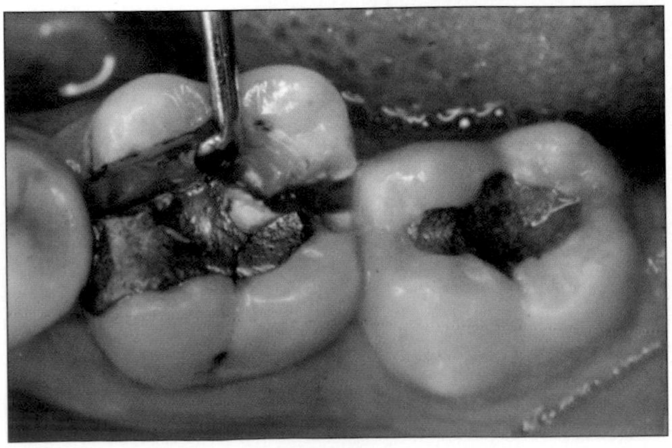

Fig. 9 Root or crown fractures can often be avoided by protecting the tooth during endodontic treatment, and providing cuspal coverage following treatment. If the tooth fractures in the vertical plane the prognosis is poor.

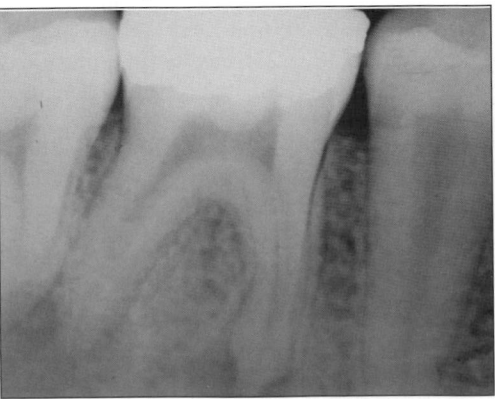

Fig. 10 Phoenix abscess. Endodontic treatment was commenced on this tooth with a chronic periradicular lesion, which had previously been symptomless. The patient returned 2 days later with extreme pain and swelling.

severe cases, it may be necessary to prescribe an antibiotic.

POST-ENDODONTIC TREATMENT

The following factors need to be considered should pain occur following sealing of the root canal system.

- High restoration
- Overfilling
- Underfilling
- Root fracture

Once obturation of the root canal space has been completed, restoration of the rest of the tooth can be carried out. The occlusion must be checked for interferences, to avoid an apical periodontitis, or worse, a fractured tooth.

Root fillings that are apparently overfilled do not as a rule cause more than mild discomfort after completion. The most likely cause of pain following obturation of the root canal space is the presence of infected material in the periapical region. The significance of an underfilled root canal is whether the canal has been properly cleaned and prepared in the first instance, and infected debris is still present in the canal. Post-endodontic pain in these circumstances may well be due to inadequate debridement of the canal.

Removal of an overextended root filling is rarely completely successful and the options left are as follows:

- Prescription of analgesics and, if the pain is more severe and infection is present, antibiotics.
- An attempt at removal of the root filling and repreparation of the root canal.
- Periradicular surgery and apicectomy.

Root fracture

The forces needed to place a satisfactory root filling, using the lateral compaction of gutta-percha technique, should not be excessive; too much pressure increases the risk of root fracture. The most common type of fracture is usually a vertical one and the prognosis is poor. Extraction, or sectioning of the root in the case of a multirooted tooth, is all that can be recommended.

1. Hasler J F, Mitchell D F. Analysis if 1628 cases of odontalgia: A corroborative study. *J Indianapolis District Dent Soc* 1963; **17**: 23–25.
2. Drinnan D L. Differential diagnosis of orofacial pain. *Dent Clin North Am* 1987; **31**: 627–643.
3. Mosaku A O, Watkins K E E, Grey N J A. The hot water test: a diagnostic procedure and a case report. *CPD Dentistry* 2000; **1**: 101–103.
4. Seltzer S, Bender I B, Zionitz M. The dynamics of pulp inflammation: Correlation between diagnostic data and histologic findings in the pulp. *Oral Surg* 1963; **16**: 846–871, 969–977.
5. Garfunkel A, Sela J, Ulmansky M. Dental pulp pathosis; clinico-pathological correlations based on 109 cases. *Oral Surg* 1973; **35**: 110–117.
6. Dummer P H, Hicks R, Huws D. Clinical signs and symptoms in pulp disease. *Int Endod J* 1980; **13**: 27–35.
7. Baumgartner J C, Mader C L. A scanning electron microscopic evaluation of four root canal irrigation systems. *J Endod* 1987; **13**: 147–157.
8. Berutti E, Marini R. A scanning electron microscopic evaluation of the debridement capability of sodium hypochlorite at different temperatures. *J Endod* 1996; **22**: 467–470.
9. Watts A, Patterson R C. The response of the mechanically exposed pulp to prednisolone and triamcinolone acetonide. *Int Endod J* 1988; **21**: 9–16.
10. Harrington GW, Natkin E. Midtreatment flare-ups. *Dent Clin North Am* 1992; **36**: 409–423.
11. Longman L P, Preston A J, Martin M V, Wilson N H. Endodontics in the adult patient: the role of antibiotics. *J Dent* 2000; **28**: 539–548.

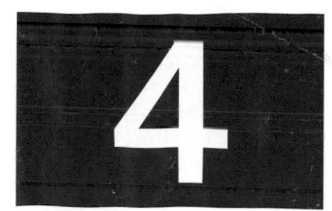

IN BRIEF
- Practitioners must be aware that the main root canals in a tooth may only provide access to the complexities of the root canal system, which must be fully cleaned of all microorganisms.
- Research has shown that the dental anatomy learned as a dental student may now be out of date.
- Knowledge of canal anatomy is essential in designing and executing access cavities that give straight line access to the main root canals.

Morphology of the root canal system

Unless the practitioner is familiar with the morphology of the roots of all teeth, and the associated intricate root canal anatomy, effective debridement and obturation may be impossible. Recent research has improved knowledge and understanding of this intricate aspect of dental practice. After studying this part you should know in what percentage of each tooth type you may expect unusual numbers of root canals and other anatomical variations.

This part may seem at first sight the most boring in the book, yet it could be the most important in improving clinical practice. Both undergraduate students and dentists on postgraduate courses frequently state that the reason they find root canal treatment so difficult, and the reason surveys frequently report inadequate treatment standards, is because they are working 'blind'. Unless a surgical microscope is available it is impossible to see down the root canal – to visualize exactly what the instruments are doing. An understanding of the architecture of the root canal system is therefore an essential prerequisite for successful root canal treatment (see Part 1, Fig. 1). As long ago as 1925, when Hess and Zurcher first published their study,[1] it became clear that teeth had complicated root canal systems rather than the simplified canals that had been previously described.

Sadly their work, and many similar publications, have largely been overlooked and dentists still remain obsessed with the concept of a 'root canal', a hollow tube down a root which has to be cleaned and shaped, eventually appearing as a nice white line on the post-operative radiograph. Undergraduate students learn the number of canals in each tooth by rote. However, many teeth have more than one canal, as described in this part. Where two canals exist within the same root, for example the mesial root of a lower molar, lateral communication (anastomosis) in the form of fins or accessory canals, occurs between them. Even roots with a single canal will have lateral and accessory canals leaving the main canal. Unless this concept of an entire root canal system is clearly understood, and a method of cleaning and shaping this system employed to address these anastomoses as well as the main canals, infection will remain in the root canal system, and the treatment may fail.

ROOT CANAL SYSTEM

The pulp chamber in the coronal part of a tooth consists of a single cavity with projections (pulp horns) into the cusps of the tooth (Fig. 1). With age, there is a reduction in the size of the chamber due to the formation of secondary dentine, which can be either physiological or pathological in origin. Reparative or tertiary dentine may be formed as a response to pulpal irritation and is irregular and less uniform in structure.

The entrances (orifices) to the root canals are to be found on the floor of the pulp chamber, usually below the centre of the cusp tips. In cross-section, the canals are ovoid, having their greatest diameter at the orifice or just below it. In longitudinal section, the canals are broader bucco-lingually than in the mesiodistal plane. The canals taper towards the apex, following the external outline of the root. The narrowest part of the canal is to be found at the 'apical constriction', which then opens out as the apical foramen and exits to one side between 0.5 and 1.0 mm from the anatomical apex. Deposition of secondary cementum may place the apical foramen as much as 2.0 mm from the anatomical apex. It must be realized, however, that the concept of a 'single' root canal with a

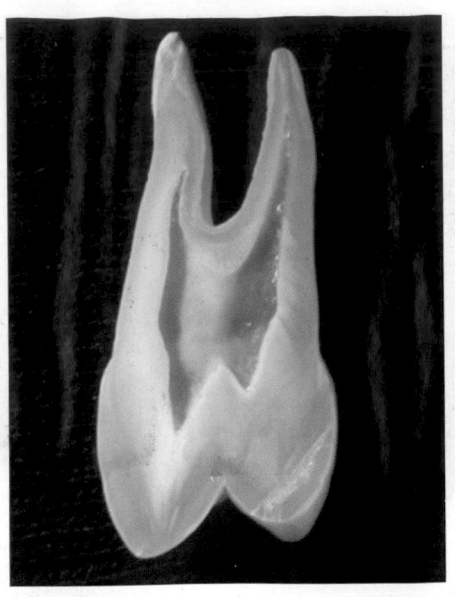

Fig. 1 The pulp chamber in the coronal part of the tooth consists of a single cavity with projections (pulp horns) into the cusps of the tooth.

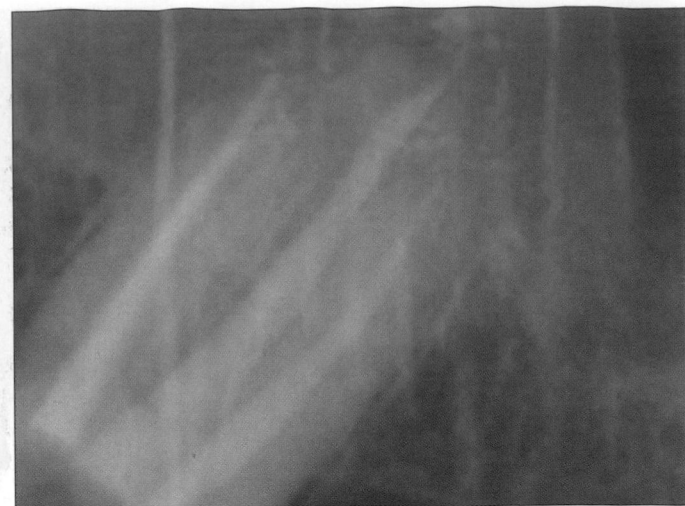

Fig. 2 The small canals found in the apical few millimetres and forming the apical delta are seen here filled with sealer.

'single' apical foramen is mistaken. The root canal may end in a delta of small canals, and during root canal treatment cleaning techniques should be employed to address this clinical situation.

LATERAL AND ACCESSORY CANALS

As previously discussed, lateral canals form channels of communication between the main body of the root canal and the periodontal ligament space. They arise anywhere along its length, at right angles to the main canal. The term 'accessory' is usually reserved for the small canals found in the apical few millimetres and forming the apical delta (Fig. 2). Both lateral and accessory canals develop due to a break in 'Hertwig's epithelial root sheath' or, during development, the sheath grows around existing blood vessels. Their significance lies in their relatively high prevalence, Kasahara *et al.*[2] finding 60% of central incisors with accessory canals, and 45% with apical foramina distant from the actual tooth apex. Kramer found that the diameter of some lateral canals was often wider than the apical constriction.[3] Lateral canals are impossible to instrument and can only be cleaned by effective irrigation with a suitable antimicrobial solution. Consequently, sealing such canals is only moderately successful.

The following descriptions of normal canal morphology and access cavities are illustrated in Figure 3 (maxilliary) and Figure 4 (mandibular).

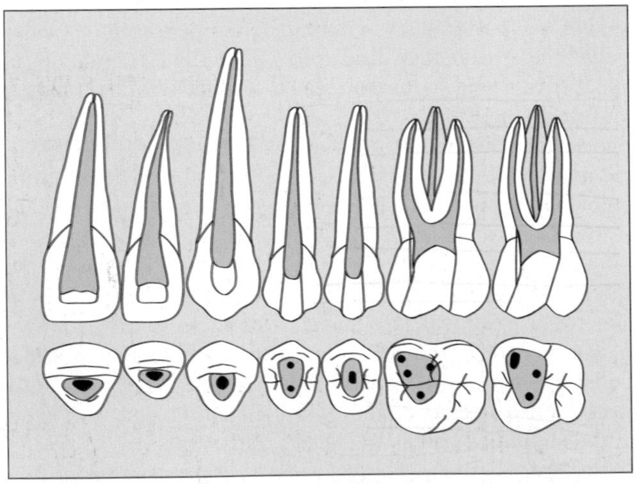

MAXILLARY CENTRAL INCISORS

These teeth almost always have one canal. When viewed on radiographs the canal appears to be fairly straight and tapering, but labiopalatally the canal will tend to curve either towards the labial or palatal aspect at about the apical third level. One feature to note is the slight narrowing of the lumen at the cervical level, which immediately opens up into the main body of the canal. The inverted-triangular shaped access cavity is cut with its base at the cingulum to give straight line access.

MAXILLARY LATERAL INCISOR

Similar in shape to the central incisors, but fractionally shorter, the apical third tends to curve distally and the canal is often very fine with thin walls. Labiopalatally, the canal is similar to the central incisor, but there is often a narrowing of the canal at the apical third level. The root is more palatally placed, an important point when any periradicular surgical procedures are carried out on this tooth. The access cavity is similar to the central incisor.

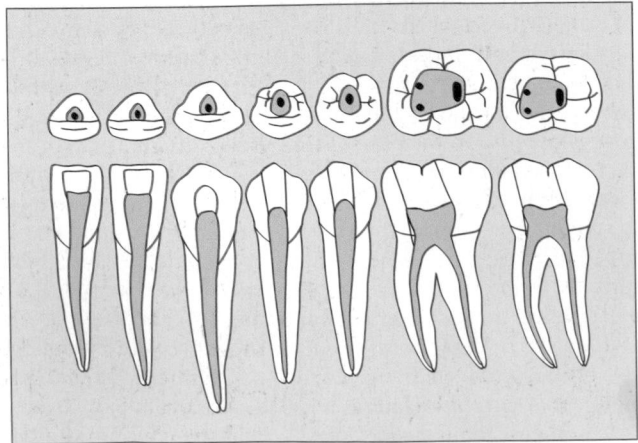

Fig. 3 The basic pulp canal shape and suggested access cavity openings in the maxilliary teeth.

Fig. 4 The basic pulp canal shape and suggested access cavity openings in the mandibular teeth.

MAXILLARY CANINE

As well as being the longest tooth in the mouth, its oval canal often seems very spacious during instrumentation. However, there is usually a sudden narrowing at the apical 2–3 mm; this leads to a danger of overinstrumentation if too large a file is used at this level. The length of this tooth can be difficult to determine on radiographs, as the apex tends to curve labially and the tooth will appear to be shorter than it actually is. The oval shape of the root canal is reflected in the shape of the access cavity.

MAXILLARY FIRST PREMOLAR

Typically, this tooth has two roots with two canals. In many ways this is the most difficult tooth to treat, as it can have a complex canal system. Variations range from one to three roots, (Fig. 5), but there are nearly always at least two canals present, even if they exit through a common apical foramen. The roots of these teeth are very delicate and at the apical third they may curve quite sharply buccally, palatally, mesially or distally, so instrumentation needs to be carried out with great care (Fig. 6). In a small percentage of cases the buccal root may subdivide into two canals in the apical third, as shown in Figure 7. An oval access cavity is cut between the cusp tips, being wider buccopalatally than mesiodistally.

MAXILLARY SECOND PREMOLAR

In 40% of cases, this tooth, which is similar in length to the first premolar, has one root with a single canal. Two canals may be found in about 58% of cases.[4] The configuration of the two canals may vary with two separate canals and two exits, two canals and one common exit, one canal dividing and having two exits. In one study,[5] it was found that 59% of maxillary second premolars had accessory canals. As with the first maxillary premolar, the apical third of the root may curve quite considerably, mainly to the distal, sometimes buccally. The access cavity is similar to the first premolar.

MAXILLARY FIRST MOLAR

This tooth has three roots. The palatal root is the longest, with an average length of 22 mm; the mesiobuccal and distobuccal roots are slightly shorter, at 21 mm average length. The percentage of mesiobuccal roots having two canals reported in the literature has increased steadily as research techniques have developed. *In vitro* studies have usually reported a higher incidence than *in vivo* studies. Stropko, reporting an extensive *in vivo* study,[6] found second canals in 73% of cases before the use of an operating microscope, but 93% following its use. The canals of the mesiobuccal root are often very fine and difficult to negotiate; consequently, more errors in instrumentation occur in this tooth than in almost any other. Anastomosis between these two canals may take the form of narrow canals or wide fins, both almost impossible to instrument. The curvature of the roots

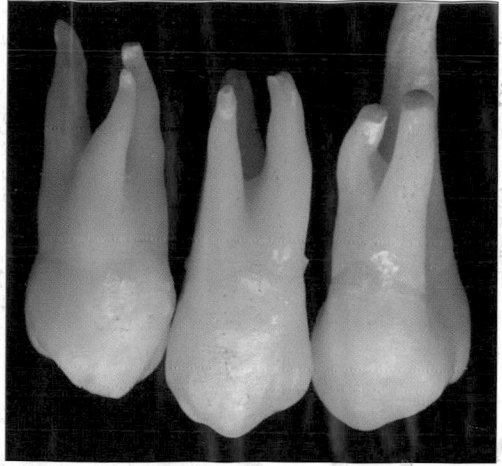

Fig. 5 Examples of upper premolars with three roots.

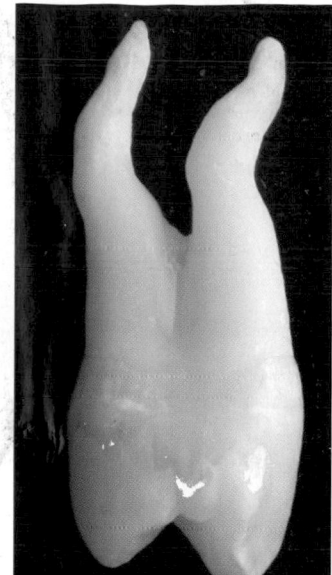

Fig. 6 The roots of upper first premolars are very delicate and may curve quite sharply buccally, palatally, mesially or distally, so instrumentation needs to be carried out with great care.

can be difficult to visualize from radiographs, and the second mesiobuccal canal is nearly always superimposed on the primary mesiobuccal canal. The palatal root has a tendency to curve towards the buccal and the apparent length on a radiograph will be shorter than its actual length. The access cavity represents the shape of the pulp chamber, enlarged slightly, and flared up on to the mesiobuccal aspect of the occlusal surface to accommodate the angle of instrument approach when working at the back of the mouth.

MAXILLARY SECOND MOLAR

This tooth is similar to the first maxillary molar, but slightly smaller and shorter, with straighter

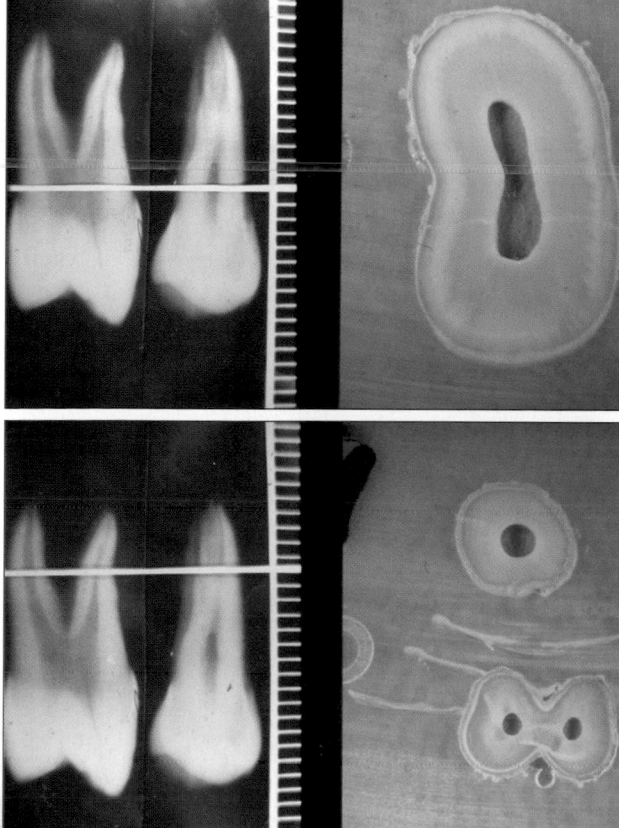

Fig. 7 Cross-sections taken at different levels in a maxillary first premolar showing the division of the buccal canal.

Fig. 8 Lower canines may occasionally be found with two separate roots.

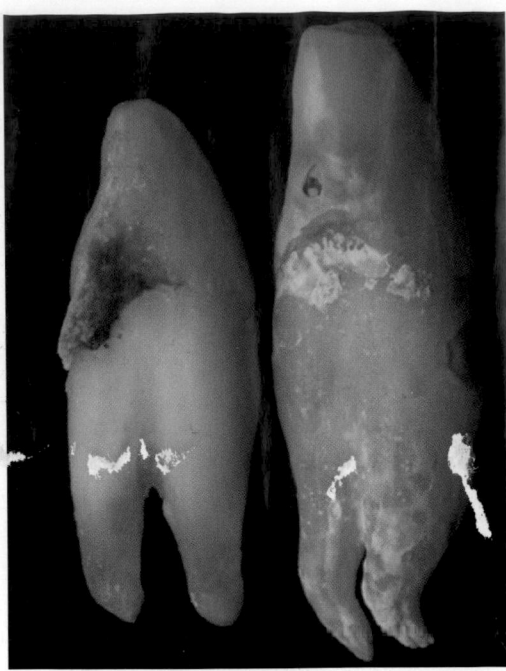

Fig. 9 A lower second premolar with a severe distal curve at the apex.

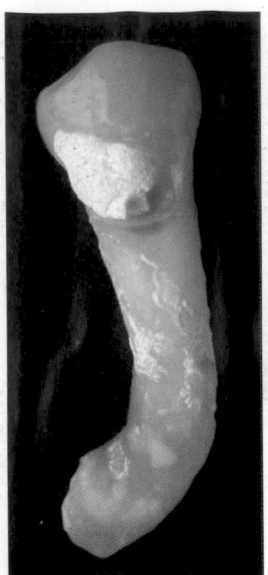

Table 1 Average root canal configurations

Tooth	Average Length	No. of roots	No. of canals
Maxillary anteriors			
Central incisor	22.5 mm	1	1
Lateral incisor	22.0 mm	1	1
Canine	26.5 mm	1	1
Maxillary premolar			
First premolar	20.6 mm	2-3	1 (6.%)
			2 (95%)
			3 (1%)
Second premolar	21.5 mm	1-3	1 (75%)
			2 (24%)
			3 (1%)
Maxillary molars			
First molar	20.8 mm	3	4 (93%)
			3 (7%)
Second molar	20.0 mm	3	4 (37%)
			3 (63%)
Third molar	17.0 mm	1-3	
Mandibular anteriors			
Central incisor	20.7 mm	1	1 (58%)
			2 (42%)
Lateral incisor	20.7 mm	1-2	1 (58%)
			2 (42%)
Canine	25.6 mm	1	1 (94%)
			2(6%)
Mandibular premolars			
First premolar	21.6 mm	1	1 (73%)
			2 (27%)
Second premolar	22.3 mm	1	1 (85%)
			2 (15%)
Mandibular molars			
First molar	21.0 mm	2-3	3 (67%)
			4 (33%)
Second molar	19.8 mm	2	2 (13%)
			3 (79%)
			4 (8%)
Third molar	18.5 mm	1-2	

roots and thinner walls. Usually there are only three canals and the roots are sometimes fused. The access cavity is the same as for the first molar, modified further to accommodate the angle of approach.

MAXILLARY THIRD MOLAR
The morphology of this tooth can vary considerably, ranging from a copy of the first or second maxillary molar to a canal system that is quite complex. They are best explored with a wide access cavity and direct vision of the individual canal anatomy.

MANDIBULAR CENTRAL AND LATERAL INCISORS
The morphology of these two teeth is very similar. The central incisor has an average length of 20.5 mm and the lateral is a little longer with an average length of 21 mm. Over 40% of these teeth have two canals, but only just over 1% have two separate foramina. Careful reading of the pre-operative radiograph may show a change in the radiodensity of the root canal, indicating division into two separate canals, and a correctly designed access cavity will facilitate checking for a second canal. This is oval in shape, commencing above the cingulum and almost notching the lingual incisal edge.

MANDIBULAR CANINE
This tooth is similar to its opposite number, although not as long. On rare occasions, two roots may exist and this can cause difficulty with instrumentation (Fig. 8). An oval access cavity is again indicated.

MANDIBULAR FIRST PREMOLAR
The canal configuration of this tooth can be quite complex. Vertucci[7] has shown that the single canal normally found may divide into two

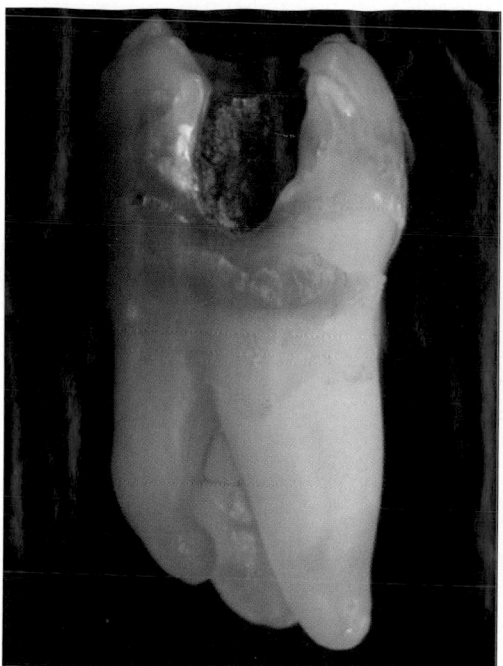

Fig. 10 Lower first molars may occasionally be found with two separate distal roots.

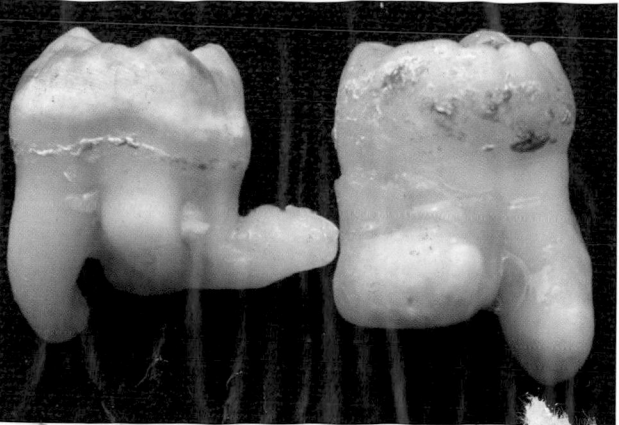

Fig. 11 The developmental anatomy of lower third molars may be quite bizarre.

MANDIBULAR SECOND MOLAR

This tooth is similar to the mandibular first molar, although a little more compact. The mesial canals tend to lie much closer together, and the incidence of two canals distally is much less. This tooth seems to be more susceptible to vertical fracture. Occasionally, the root canals may join in a buccal fin giving a 'C-shaped' canal, which may lead all the way to the apex.[10] The access cavity is similar to that of the first molar.

MANDIBULAR THIRD MOLAR

Together with the maxillary third molar, this tooth displays some of the most irregular canal configurations to be found in the adult dentition, as seen in Figure 11. However, the mesial inclination of the tooth generally makes access easier. The canal orifices are not too difficult to locate, but the degree of curvature of the apical half of the root canal system is often pronounced. Added to this, the apex is frequently poorly developed and lies close to the inferior alveolar canal. A large access cavity allowing direct visualization of the floor of the pulp chamber enables the canal orifices to be identified.

It should always be remembered that whilst the above descriptions are the norm, occasionally other teeth may be encountered with unusual or even bizarre anatomy. This may only be discovered after the treatment has failed and the tooth has been extracted. Clues may sometimes be found by careful examination of the radiographs, especially with the use of magnification, as described in Part 5.

canals and two apical foramina in 25% of cases. It is the way in which the second canal branches that can cause difficulty with instrumentation. Occasionally, the canal terminates with an extensive delta, making obturation of the accessory canals even more challenging. As in the upper premolars, the access cavity is oval between the cusp tips.

MANDIBULAR SECOND PREMOLAR

This tooth is similar to the first premolar, except that the incidence of a second canal is very much lower. One study stated this to be 12%.[7] Another study revealed that only 2.5% had two apical foramina.[8] Consequently, it is a much easier tooth to treat compared with the mandibular first premolar, unless the radiograph reveals a sharp distal curve at the apex as shown in the extracted tooth at Figure 9.

MANDIBULAR FIRST MOLAR

This is often the most heavily restored tooth in the adult dentition and seems to be a frequent candidate for root canal treatment. Generally there are two roots and three canals: two canals in the mesial root and one large oval canal distally. According to Skidmore and Bjorndal,[9] one third of these molars have four canals. Occasionally, three roots are to be found: usually two distal and one mesial (Fig. 10), rarely one distal and two mesial. Anastomoses occur between the canals and accessory communication with the furcation area is a frequent finding. The mesiobuccal canal tends to exhibit the greatest degree of curvature. The access cavity once again represents the shape of the pulp chamber, enlarged slightly, and flared up on to the mesiobuccal aspect of the occlusal surface to accommodate the angle of instrument approach when working at the back of the mouth.

1. Hess W, Zurcher E. *The anatomy of the root canals of the teeth of the permanent dentition and the anatomy of the root canals of the deciduous dentition and the first permanent molars.* London: Basle, Sons and Danielson, 1925.
2. Kasahara E, Yasuda E, Yamamoto A, Anzai M. Root canal systems of the maxillary central incisor. *J Endod* 1990; **16**: 158–161.
3. Kramer I R. The vascular architecture of the human dental pulp. *Arch Oral Biol* 1960; **2**: 177–189.
4. Bellizi R, Hartwell G. Radiographic evaluation of root canal anatomy of *in vivo* endodontically treated maxillary premolars. *J Endod* 1985; **11**: 37–39.
5. Vertucci F J, Seeling A, Gillis R. Root canal morphology of the human maxillary second premolar. *Oral Surg* 1974; **38**: 456–464.
6. Stropko J J. Canal morphology of maxillary molars: clinical observations of canal configurations. *J Endod* 1999; **25**: 446–450.

7. Zillich R, Dowson J. Root canal morphology of the mandibular first and second premolars. *Oral Surg* 1973; 36: 738–744.

8. Vertucci F J. Root canal morphology of mandibular premolars. *J Am Dent Assoc* 1978; 97: 47–50.

9. Skidmore A E, Bjorndal A M. Root canal morphology of the human mandibular first molar. *Oral Surg* 1971; 32: 778–784.

10. Melton D C, Krall K V, Fuller M W. Anatomical and histological features of C-shaped canals in mandibular second molars. *J Endod* 1991; 17: 384–388.

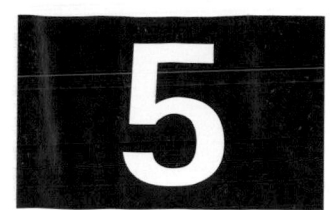
IN BRIEF
- A basic pack of all the endodontic instruments required must be available suitably sterilised to ensure rapid efficient treatment.
- Modern radiographic techniques facilitate swift diagnosis and treatment procedures.
- The development of endodontic instruments from reamers to greater taper nickel titanium files is considered.
- The importance of thorough and efficient irrigation with appropriate antiseptic agents is discussed, together with the necessary precautions.

Basic instruments and materials for root canal treatment

In this part the basic endodontic instruments necessary for effective root canal treatment are described. The properties of, and manufacturer's claims for, new instruments and techniques may be compared to these basic principles before they are purchased and introduced to clinical practice. Having the correct instruments for different clinical situations may make treatment both more efficient and more effective.

Many dental practitioners find it difficult to resist new gadgets, and there are an inordinate number made specifically for endodontics. New instruments and materials are frequently sold with the promise of simplifying a technique, shortening the time taken or even increasing the success rate. Unfortunately, these promises are often not fulfilled, and the result may be cupboards in the practice containing unwanted endodontic armamentaria. It would be impossible to cover all the instruments and materials used in endodontics in one part, but it is hoped to mention most of the basic equipment and discuss some of the newer items. For continuity, some instruments will be described in the relevant parts. The majority of the instruments and materials referred to in this part are generic, and may be purchased from most dental supply companies.

INSTRUMENT PACK

A basic pack of instruments must be available specifically for routine root canal procedures. An example is given in Figure 1. A front surface reflecting mouth mirror is preferable to prevent the double image of the fine detail in an access cavity that occurs with a conventional mirror. Endolocking tweezers allow small items to be gripped safely and passed between nurse and operator. A DG16 endodontic probe is required to detect canal orifices. The excavator is long shanked, with a small blade to allow access into the pulp chamber. The pocket-measuring probe is useful, a routine CPITN probe with clearly vis-

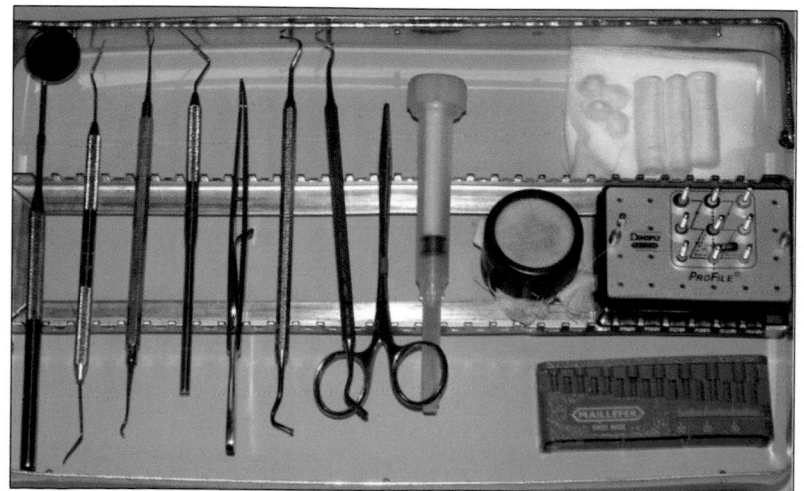

Fig. 1 An endodontic instrument pack. From left to right; front surface reflecting mirror; DG16 endodontic probe; Western probe; CPITN probe; endo–locking tweezers; long shank excavator; flat plastic, artery forceps, endodontic syringe; plus clean stand, file stand, measuring device, sterile cotton wool rolls and pledgets.

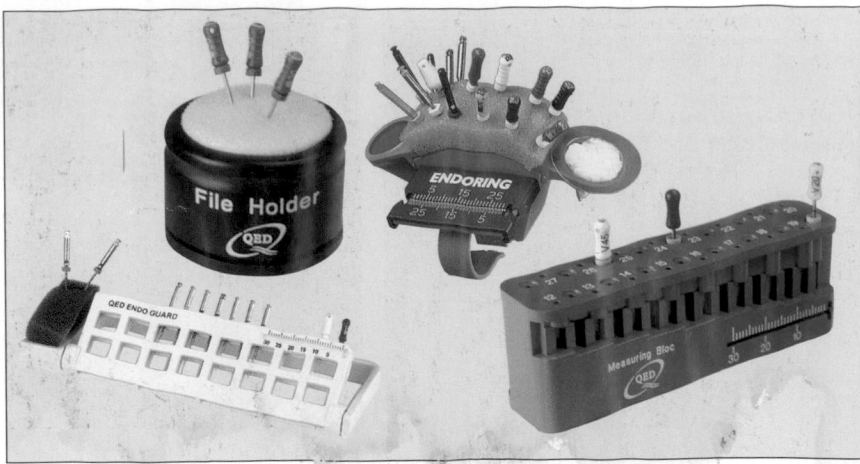

Fig. 2 A selection of file holders.

Fig. 4 The rubber dam equipment; clamps, dental floss, forceps, sheet, punch, frame and napkin.

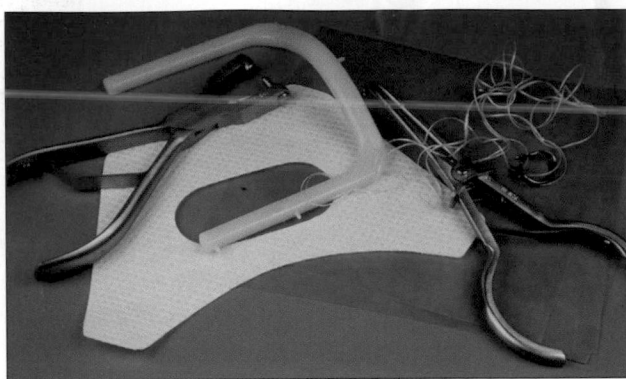

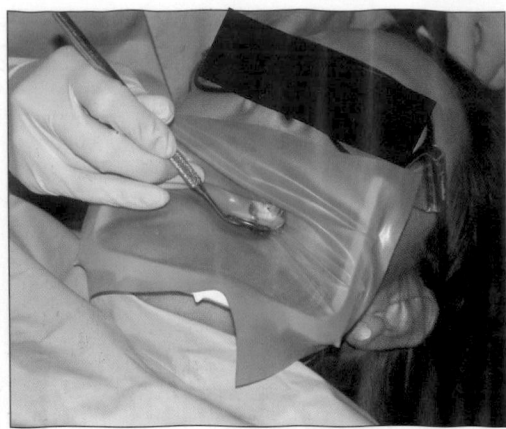

Fig. 3 A patient wearing safety glasses, a waterproof protective bib and a rubber dam.

RUBBER DAM

Rubber dam is essential in root canal treatment for three reasons:

- To provide an operating field free from oral contamination.
- To prevent the patient swallowing or inhaling root canal instruments or medicaments.
- To give good visual access by retracting the lips and tongue.

A basic kit for rubber dam equipment is shown in Figure 4. Details of this equipment, and of the techniques for the application of rubber dam, are given in the next part.

RADIOGRAPHIC EQUIPMENT

Long-cone parallel radiography is a requirement for endodontics,[1] because it gives an undistorted view of the teeth and surrounding structures and is repeatable, thus allowing more accurate assessment of periapical healing. The bisecting angle technique should no longer be employed. It is further recommended that rectangular collimation

ible gradations is ideal. A furcation probe is useful to check for the presence of furcation involvement. Other items usually included are a flat plastic, sterile cotton wool rolls, sterile cotton wool pledgets, artery forceps to grip a periapical radiograph and a metal ruler, or other measuring device that may be sterilized. A clean-stand or other device such as the endoring is required to hold the endodontic instruments. Paper points are also required, and the simplest method of storage and use is to purchase presterilized packs with five points in each pack.

These instruments should be sterile when treatment commences, and every possible effort must be made to avoid contamination. Few practices will have an autoclave sufficiently large to take a metal tray with a lid that may contain an entire set of sterile instruments. If an open tray system is used, as illustrated in Figure 1, it is useful to have all endodontic instruments in sterilized containers, such as the clean stand or endodontic ring shown in Figure 2. This allows the instruments to be easily controlled, and accessed by both the operator and assistant during treatment.

PATIENT PROTECTION

Glasses are needed to protect the patient's eyes. Figure 3 also shows a waterproof bib being worn, as the patient's clothes must be protected against accidental spillage of sodium hypochlorite, a frequent source of patient complaint or even litigation.

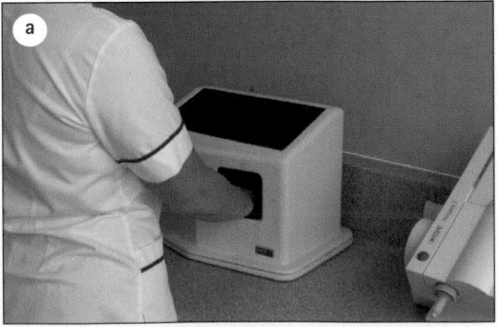

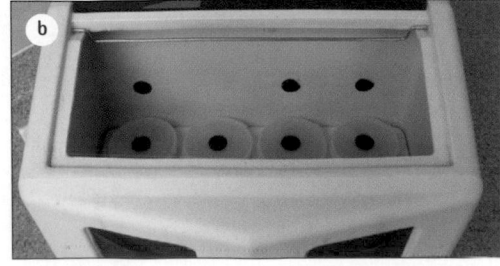

Fig. 6 a) A manual radiographic processing unit being used and b) containing rapid developing and fixing chemicals.

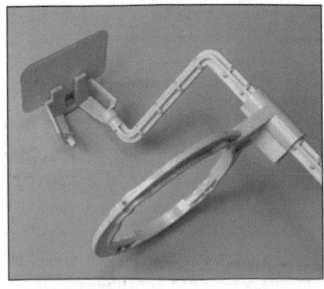

Fig. 5 A film holder for taking parallel radiographs, incorporating a cage device to fit over the rubber dam clamp.

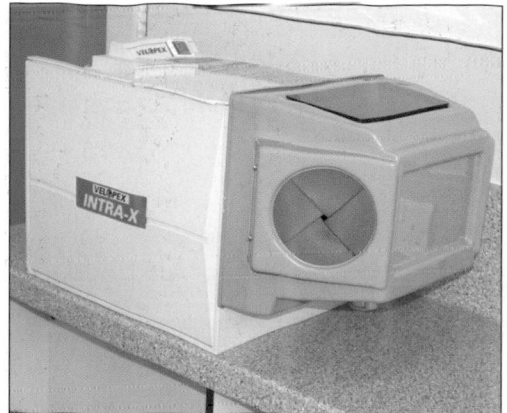

Fig. 7 An automatic radiographic processor, with a simple device to bypass the drying cycle.

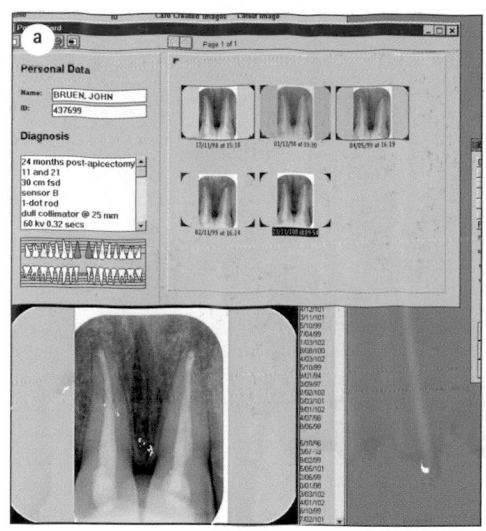

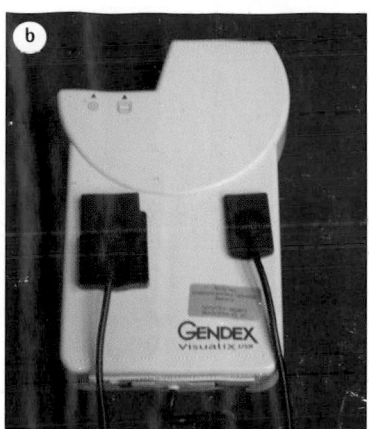

Fig. 8 An illustration of the computer screen produced by digital radiography, enabling immediate viewing and manipulation of the image The sensor plate or 'film' may be either loose, resembling a conventional periapical radiographic film, which must be inserted into the machine for processing, or linked by cable to the processor as in b).

be fitted on all new radiographic equipment, and retro-fitted to existing equipment as soon as possible. There are many beam-aiming devices available to hold the x-ray film parallel to the tooth. Figure 5 shows an example of a popular holder, with a special cage attachment to fit over a rubber dam clamp.

A quick, reliable method of viewing radiographic images is essential for endodontics. Considerable time can be lost if such a system is not available, especially on those occasions when the exposed film does not show the required detail. Practitioners using conventional radiography may wish to purchase an x-ray film processor with rapid developing and fixing solutions, capable of producing a radiograph for viewing in under a minute; an example is shown in Figure 6. However, a modern automatic processor (Fig. 7) may be adjusted to deliver wet films in under two minutes. Films from both types of processor should be carefully dried after viewing for accurate storage in the patient's records.

A modern alternative involves the use of digital radiography. A sensor plate, appropriately sterilized and scaled, is used in place of the conventional film. The sensor may be either directly linked to the computer, or resemble a conventional periapical film packet. The resultant image is digitally processed and projected upon the computer screen in a matter of seconds. The quality of the image can be manipulated to enable greater clarity when reading the picture. For purposes of record keeping, the image may be either dated, labelled and stored in the central database, or a hard copy printed for the patient's records. An example of such a system, and the images produced, is shown in Figure 8.

The pre-operative radiograph contains much information to assist the operator, which may not be seen if the film is carelessly viewed. An x-ray viewer and some form of magnification are needed to examine periapical films, and it is very helpful if glare from the light around the radiograph can be excluded (Fig. 9).

DEVELOPMENT OF HAND INSTRUMENTS
For many years the standard cutting instruments have been the reamer, K-type file and Hedstroem

file. These root canal preparation instruments have been manufactured to a size and type advised by the International Standards Organisation (ISO). The specifications recommended are complex and differ according to the type of instrument. For most standardized instruments the number refers to its diameter at the tip in one hundredths of a millimetre; a number 10, for example, means that it has a tip diameter of 0.10 mm. Colour coding originally denoted the size, but now represents a sequence of sizes. All these instruments have a standard 2% taper over their working length.

Recent changes in both metallurgy and endodontic concepts have led to the introduction of a range of new instruments which do not conform to these specifications. These are described individually later and in Part 7. These instruments have been widely adopted, and appear to give consistently better results in root canal treatment. However, the conventional 2% taper instruments are essential for the initial exploration of most root canals, for difficult procedures such as bypassing separated instruments, and for the apical preparation of some difficult canals.

Conventional 'standardized' instruments are made of steel, which may wear quickly in dentine, and small size files may be regarded as disposable. Although some hand files are now available in a nickel–titanium alloy, which is more resistant to wear than ordinary steel, the increased cost and inability to pre-curve has not led to their widespread use. The majority of these modern files are manufactured with a modified non-aggressive tip to prevent iatrogenic damage to the canal system, and improve performance of the instrument. Figure 10 shows the different appearance of the principal types of these instruments.

K–type file
These instruments were originally made from a square or triangular blank, machine twisted to form a tight spiral. The angle of the blades or flutes is consequently near a right-angle to the shank, so that either a reaming or a filing action

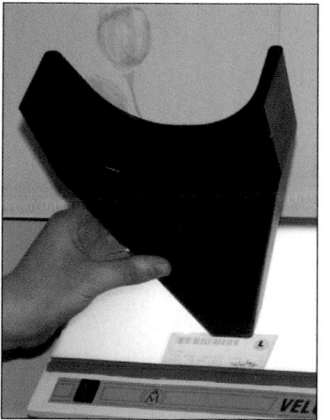

Fig. 9 A radiographic viewer designed to eliminate extraneous light and magnify the image.

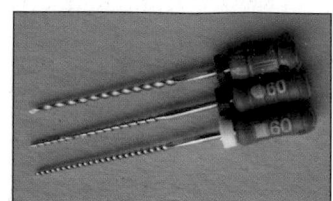

Fig. 10 Conventional hand instruments; top – reamer with red stop; middle – Hedstroem file with black stop; bottom – K-flex file with yellow stop.

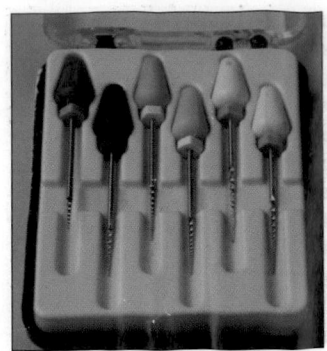

Fig. 11 A pack of hand files of greater taper, 12% taper (blue), 10% (red), 8% (yellow) and 6% (white).

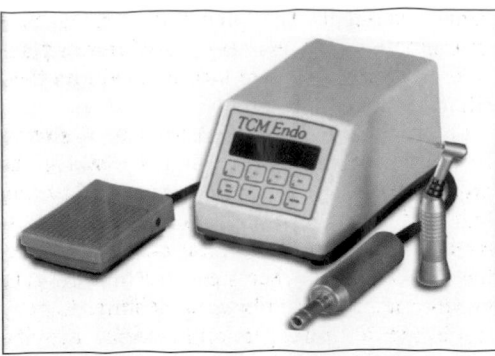

Fig. 12 A low-speed, high-torque motor required for use with nickel-titanium rotary instruments.

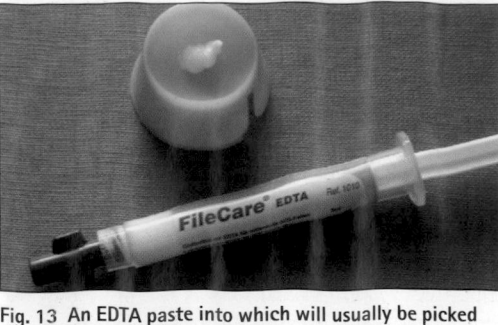

Fig. 13 An EDTA paste into which will usually be picked up on each instrument before use.

may be used. The K-type file has been subject to continuous development. The K-flex file is made from a rhomboid or diamond shaped blank. The acute angle of this shape provides the instrument with two sharp blades and the narrower diameter allows greater flexibility in the shaft than a conventional K-file. The manufacturers claim that more debris is collected between the blades and therefore removed from the canal than with a standard K-file. The Flex-o-file employs a more flexible type of steel. It does not fracture easily and is so flexible that it is possible to tie a knot in the shank of the smaller sizes.

The latest developments in file design have seen a move away from the ISO standard 2% taper to files with increasing tapers of up to 12%, made in a nickel-titanium alloy. Although most of these new developments are used with an electric motor, hand files of greater taper are available. These are illustrated in Figure 11. Their use is described in Part 7.

Although most K-type files were originally used with an 'in-out' circumferential filing technique, the 'balanced-force' technique, described in Part 7, is now considered the manipulation method of choice.

Hedstroem file

The Hedstroem file is machined from a round tapered blank. A spiral groove is cut into the shank, producing a sharp blade. Only a true filing action should be used with this instrument because of the angle of the blade. There is a strong possibility of fracture if a reaming action is used and the blades are engaged in the dentine. The Hedstroem file is useful for removing gutta-percha root fillings.

Other hand files

Different types of hand file have been introduced from time to time with varied structure and cutting action. The Unifile and Helifile were modifications of the Hedstroem design. The Mani Flare file is made from a triangular blank, and features a greater taper than conventional 2% files. It is essential when considering the use of new file designs that the operator understands the basic principles of canal preparation, and compares and contrasts the properties with the file manipulation technique currently being used.

Reamer

The reamer is constructed from a square or triangular blank, machine twisted into a spiral but with fewer cutting flutes than a file. The reamer will only cut dentine when it is rotated in the canal; the mode of action described for its use is a quarter to a half turn to cut dentine, and withdrawal to remove the debris. The stiffness of an instrument increases with each larger size, so that larger reamers in curved canals will tend to cut a wider channel near the apical end of the root canal (apical zipping). Considerable damage may be caused to a root canal by the incorrect use of a reamer, and their routine use is no longer recommended.

Power-assisted instruments

Handpieces providing a mechanical movement to the root canal cutting instrument have been available since 1964. Their function was primarily a reciprocating action through 90° and/or a vertical movement, according to the design and make. Because steel files do not have the flexibility necessary for rotary movements in a curved canal without damaging the canal configuration, these instruments were never really acceptable in endodontic practice.

A totally new concept in canal preparation came with the development of sonic and ultrasonically activated endodontic handpieces. Much research took place into the mode of action and effectiveness of these machines. It was generally agreed that while the sonic machines were more effective at hard tissue removal, the ultrasonic machines were more effective in irrigation. The piezo-electric machines were found to be more effective than the magnetostrictive. The latter also generated more heat, and irrigation with effective quantities of sodium hypochlorite was found to be difficult.

The ultrasonic action causes acoustic microstreaming of the irrigant, intensive circular fluid movement carried right to the tip of the instrument, found to be very effective at canal debridement. This effect is reduced, however, when the file is constrained by the canal wall. The main use of these instruments today is in irrigation and debridement, using a freely oscillating file in a sodium hypochlorite filled canal, after thorough mechanical canal shaping.[2]

However, the development of nickel-titanium alloy for endodontic instruments has allowed the concept of an engine driven endodontic instrument to be fully explored. The total flexibility of this alloy, and the use of radial lands on the cutting flutes to keep the instrument centred in the canal, permit controlled cutting of the dentine walls. Most major manufacturers have developed a nickel-titanium rotary system. Lightspeed, Profiles, GT Rotary files, FlexMaster, Quantec system, Hero, K3, Protaper, and no doubt more will appear before this book is even published. It would not be possible to describe each of these fully, but the basic concepts are presented here, with a general description of their use being given in Part 7.

The systems will generally conform to one of three patterns.

- The system may have a standard ISO tip size sequence, with the instruments being manufactured with an increased taper, usually either 4% or 6%.

- The system may be presented with a single tip size, but with the sequence of file sizes having an increased taper of up to 12%. In order to accommodate this taper in a narrow root canal, the diameter of the instrument is usually limited to 1 mm, giving quite a short functional blade in the greater tapers.

- Both of these new developments may be combined into one system.

A low-speed, controlled-torque motor is necessary when using these instruments, as illustrated in Figure 12.

Irrigation and lubrication materials

It is generally accepted in endodontic practice that sodium hypochlorite is the most suitable solution for irrigation of the root canal system. Normal household bleach is approximately 5.5% sodium hypochlorite solution, and this may be diluted with purified water up to five times to the operator's preference. Research has shown that the antibacterial effect is the same for a 0.5% and a 5.0% solution.[3] However, the greater the dilution the less effective is the solution at dissolving organic debris in the root canal system.

Great vigilance is essential when using sodium hypochlorite, and practitioners must be aware of the risks and dangers involved in its use. Irrigation under pressure may force the solution through the apical foramen into the periradicular tissues, which may result in a rapid, painful and serious inflammatory response. The patient will be extremely distressed, and little can be done to relieve the situation which may take several days to resolve. Cases have also been reported where excess pressure on the syringe has resulted in the needle coming loose and hypochlorite spraying over the patient, operator and assistant. Protective goggles are essential for the patient and all staff. Clothing should also be protected. The defence societies have received claims from irate patients for damaged clothing following root

canal treatment. The practitioner must have appropriate risk assessment procedures in place when such materials are incorporated into their clinical practice.

Chlorhexidine solution 0.2% has a similar antibacterial action, but will not dissolve the organic debris found in parts of the canal system inaccessible to hand instrumentation, such as lateral canals, fins and apical deltas. However, the substantivity associated with this irrigant means that it will adhere to dentine, thereby exhibiting a prolonged antibacterial activity. Although chlorhexidine may not be quite as effective as sodium hypochlorite, its use should not be dismissed.

Researchers are constantly seeking improved methods of cleaning root canals; reports have appeared recently relating to the use of electro-activated water as an irrigant,[4] and the use of high frequency electric current.[5] These and others may prove interesting developments in root canal preparation and irrigation.

EDTA paste (Ethylenediamine tetra-acetic acid) is a chelating agent which softens the dentine of the canal walls and greatly facilitates canal preparation (Fig 13). EDTA solution may be used as an irrigant at the end of the canal preparation phase to assist removal of the smear layer prior to placement of an intervisit dressing, or obturation.

Burs

Several types of bur may be required for root canal treatment. Some of these are described below, and shown in Figure 14.

Cutting an access cavity

It is generally accepted that high speed burs should be used to gain access and shape the cavity. A diamond or tungsten carbide tapered fissure bur is used for initial penetration of the roof of the pulp chamber. A tapered safe-ended diamond or tungsten carbide bur is then used to remove the roof of the pulp chamber without damaging the floor.

Location of canal

Burs should only be used as a last resort to locate a sclerosed canal because of the danger of perforation. Small round burs are used; the standard length is usually too short but longer shank burs are available. Specially designed ultrasonic tips may also be used to remove secondary dentine, assist in the identification of canal orifices and in shaping the canal orifice during preparation. The use of ultrasonic tips has become more widespread with the introduction of a wider range of fittings to different piezo-electronic machines. Figure 15 shows the diamond coated CPR® tips, designed for troughing and chasing sclerosed canals, and the BUC® tips, with variable grades of diamond grit for refining access cavity walls and line angles, removing obstructions and cutting around posts. As with all instruments and materials, the manufacturer's instructions and guidance should be carefully

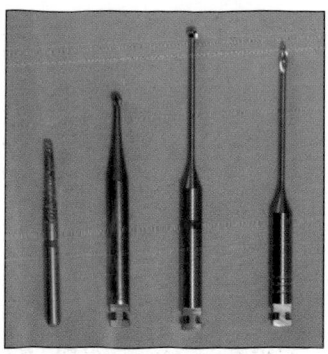

Fig. 14 Some of the burs specifically manufactured for endodontic treatment; a safe-tipped access bur; a long-shanked round bur; a swan-necked bur; a Gates-Glidden bur.

Fig. 15 (a) CPR® ultrasonic tips, now available to fit different piezo-electronic machines. (b) Also shown are KiS tips for periradicular surgery.

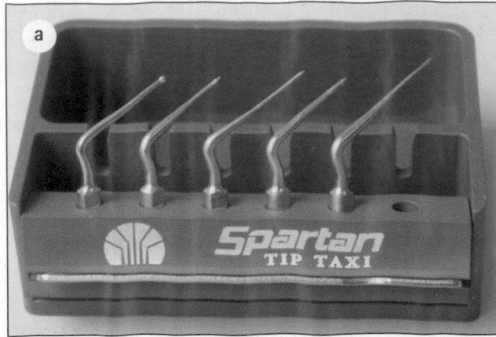

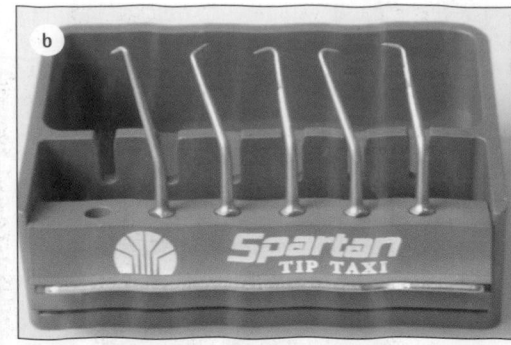

followed or these delicate diamond tips may be damaged. It is generally wise to use them with a low power setting, and to ensure that they are in contact with dentine before activating the piezo-electric unit.

Canal preparation

The use of rotary cutting instruments in a standard handpiece is condemned because of the danger of fracture of the instrument or perforation of the root canal. The exception to this rule is the Gates–Glidden bur, which has a safe-ended tip. In addition, the site of fracture, if it does occur, is almost always near the hub so the fractured piece is easily removed. In the past this bur has been recommended for initial flaring of the coronal portion of the canal. This may now be carried out in a more controlled manner with a nickel-titanium orifice shaper. The Gates–Glidden bur may also be used to make post space and to remove gutta-percha from the canal. Gates–Glidden burs are manufactured in six sizes; their use is described in Part 7.

Measurement of working length

There are two established methods of assessing the working length of a root canal: one by radiography and the other with the use of an electronic device apex locator (Fig. 16). Both methods will be described in Part 7.

Once the working length has been confirmed, the individual preparation instruments must be accurately marked to length accordingly. There are many different gadgets available for transfer of the working length; the author prefers the device shown in Figure 17. There are also different stops for the instrument, the most popular being rubber or silicone stops. These should always be placed at right angles to the shank of the instrument. Ideally the stops should be either notched, or pear shaped, so that in curved canals the notch or point of the pear may be directed towards the curve placed in the instrument.

Sterilization

Any instrument which is placed in the root canal should be sterile, for two reasons. Firstly, to prevent the introduction to the root canal system of extraneous microorganisms, which may severely compromise treatment, for example pseudomonas.[6] Secondly, if instruments and devices were to be used on different patients, to prevent cross-infection between patients. Bacte-

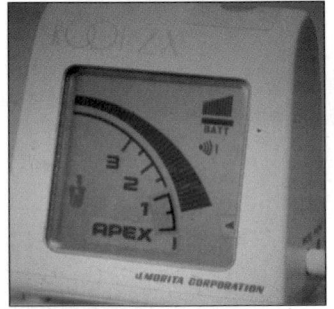

Fig. 16 An electronic apex locator.

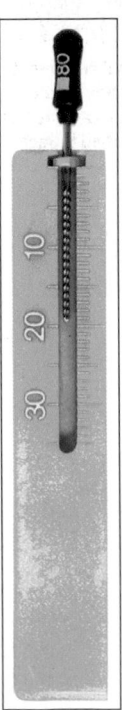

Fig. 17 A device for setting instruments at the correct working length

ria, viruses, fungi and prions may contaminate instruments and research has shown that some of these may not be destroyed by any method of sterilization.[7] Figure 18 illustrates this dramatically. Concern has been raised over the sterilization of other items of dental equipment as well.[8]

Under the Medical Devices Directive, the manufacturer of any dental instrument has an obligation to inform the end-user (ie the dentist) how their product should be decontaminated. It is essential that this guidance is followed. Whatever may be written in this and other texts may be superseded at any time. Dentists should therefore ensure that they are familiar with and conform to the manufacturer's instructions. At present, some endodontic instruments are marked with the symbol shown in Figure 19 indicating that they are single use instruments. It is assumed that all manufacturers will shortly follow this Medical Devices Directive.

It may, however, be necessary to sterilize instruments for further treatment of the same patient on a subsequent occasion when cross-infection control would not be a problem. After use, instruments must be cleaned as soon as possible to remove debris which harbours and protects microorganisms. Cleaning is carried out by scrubbing in warm water and detergent, although the debris may be first removed from most root canal instruments by stabbing them into a sponge. The best method of cleaning is to place the instruments into an ultrasonic bath. The cavitational effects of ultrasonics will dislodge debris from places which are inaccessible to normal cleaning. When the instruments are clean they must be sterilized in an autoclave. Microorganisms are destroyed at lower temperatures and in a shorter period in moist heat as all biological reactions are catalysed in water. The disadvantages of autoclaving are that metal instruments tend to corrode and sharp instruments are dulled.

Barbed broach

This instrument has sharp rasps pointing towards the handle. They may be used to remove the contents of the root canal before commencing shaping procedures. A vital pulp may be extirpated when carrying out elective endodontic procedures, or when treating a tooth with an irreversible pulpitis, by introducing the barbed broach deep in the canal, twisting it a quarter to a half turn, and withdrawing, as shown in Figure 20.

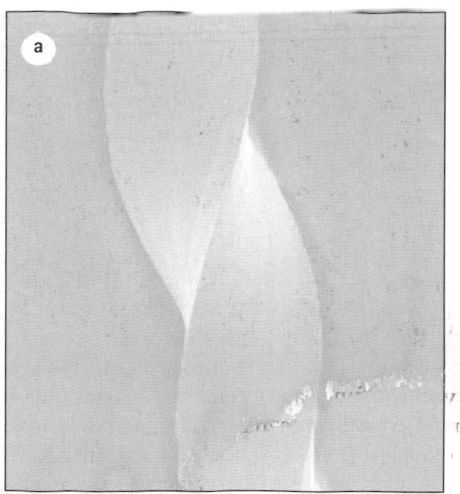
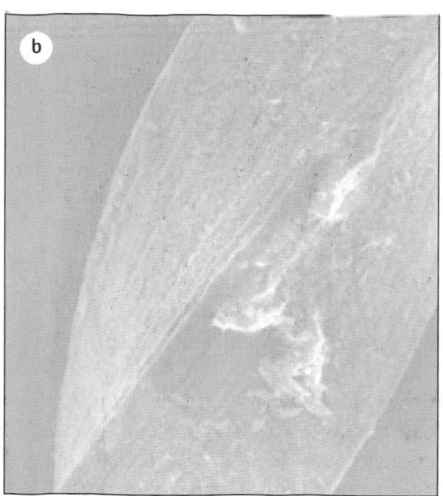
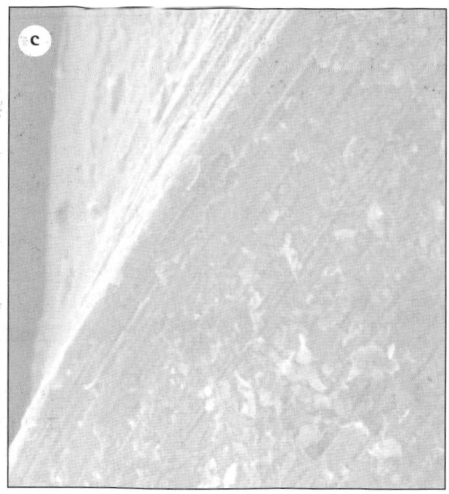

Fig. 18 Illustrations from the work on decontamination of endodontic instruments by Dr Andrew Smith, Glasgow: a) photomicrograph (x16) of an unused endodontic file; b) photomicrograph (x16) of a used instrument after sterilization; c) SEM (x500) of the file shown in illustration b.

Spiral root canal fillers

Spiral root canal fillers are seldom used in modern endodontics. Their main use is for the insertion of calcium hydroxide into the root canal. When a spiral filler is required, the blade type is preferred by the author, as this is the least likely to fracture. It is essential to ensure that the size selected fits loosely and passively to the required depth before the instrument is rotated in the root canal (Fig. 21).

ROOT CANAL FILLING MATERIALS
Gutta-percha

Gutta-percha is the most commonly used material for the obturation of the prepared root canal system. Standardized gutta-percha points correspond to the ISO sizing system with a 2% taper. Various other shapes are now available to complement the recently introduced increased taper filing systems (Fig 22). Gutta-percha is the dried resin of the Taban tree, and exists in two forms. Alpha phase is the natural form, but when heated and cooled the beta-phase results. This latter is normally used for root canal filling points.

Gutta-percha points in fact contain only about 20% gutta-percha. The major component

is zinc oxide (up to 75%), with the remainder comprising various resins, waxes and metallic sulphates to the specific manufacturer's formula.

Sealers/cements

Root canal sealers play an important role in the obturation of the prepared root canal system, as described in Part 8. Although many proprietary products are available (Fig. 23), they may generally be divided into three groups, according to their main constituents: eugenol, non-eugenol and medicated.

Eugenol

The eugenol-containing group may be divided into sealers based on the Rickert's formula (1931) and those based on Grossman's (1958) (Table 1). The essential difference between the two groups is that Rickert's contains precipitated silver and Grossman's has a barium or bismuth salt as the radiopacifier. The disadvantage of Rickert's sealer is that the silver will stain dentine a dark grey. One of the most widely used sealers in this group is Tubliseal, a two-paste system and, consequently, simple to mix; it does not contain silver. Tubliseal EWT (extended working time) is preferred.

Non-eugenol sealers

Some sealers are manufactured with a calcium hydroxide base instead of zinc oxide/eugenol,

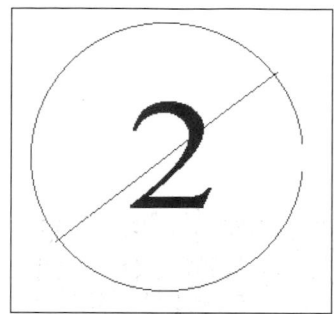

Fig. 19 The symbol indicating instruments intended for single use only.

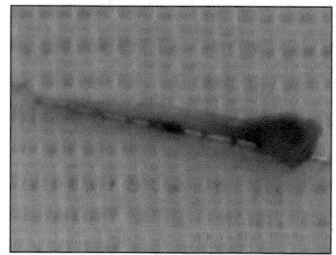

Fig. 20 During root canal treatment of a tooth diagnosed as having an irreversible pulpitis, the vital pulp has been extirpated on a barbed broach.

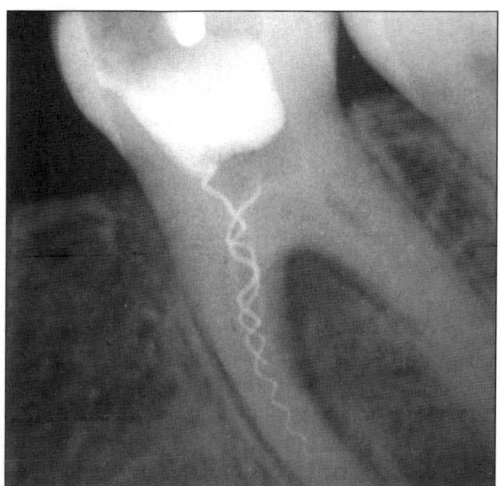

Fig. 21 Spiral fillers may fracture if the size is not verified passively before rotating in the canal.

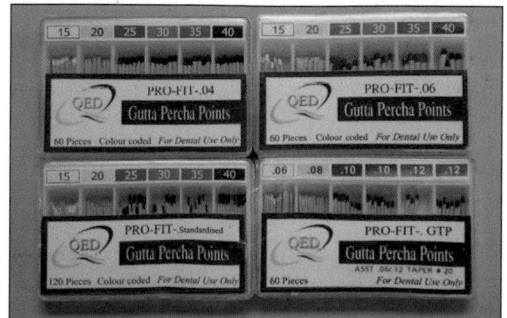

Fig. 22 Some of the different gutta–percha points: standarized; greater taper; 04 and 06 taper; feather tipped.

Fig. 23 A selection of root canal sealers.

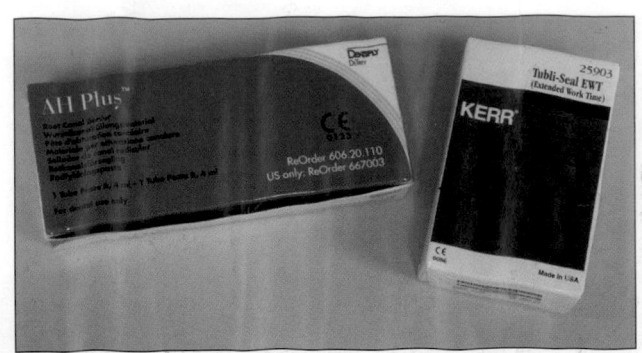

Table 1 Grossman's sealer	
Powder	
Zinc Oxide	42.0%
Staybelite resin	27.0%
Bismuth subcarbonate	15.0%
Barium sulfate	15.0%
Sodium borate (anhydrous)	1.0%
Liquid	
Eugenol	100%

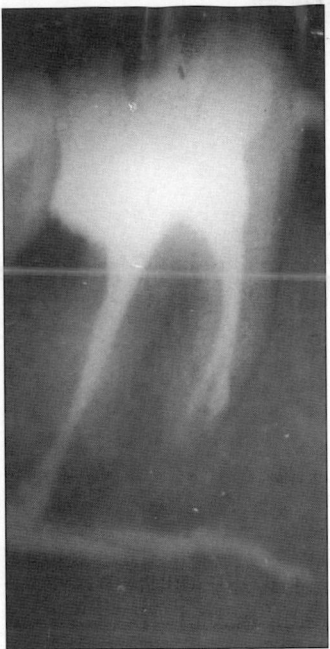

Fig. 24 A medicolegal case where a formaldehyde containing root canal sealer has been extruded into the inferior dental canal, causing paraesthesia of the lip.

for example Sealapex. This is promoted as having a therapeutic effect, although there has been little reported on this in the endodontic literature. It has been shown, however, that the calcium hydroxide is prone to leakage,[9] which may result in unwanted voids in the seal.

Other sealers are manufactured that contain a wide variety of chemicals. AH+ is an epoxy resin base with a bisphenoldiglycidyl ether liquid. It has a long working time and seals well to dentine. The original AH26 initially caused a severe inflammatory response, which subsided after some weeks, but AH+ is far more biocompatible. Diaket is a polyketone and is presented as a fine powder and thick viscous liquid. The setting time is 8 minutes on the mixing pad and somewhat quicker in the root canal. A glass ionomer cement, Ketac-Endo, is available, which has a relatively low toxicity.

A more recent addition to this group is Roekoseal, a silicone polymer. Although initial experience of this material is favourable, there has been little published on several of these recent materials, and the prudent clinician may wish to await the results of extended clinical trials before adopting these into their practice.

Medicated

The current thinking is that provided the principles of root canal preparation and filling are observed, there is no justification for the use of therapeutic sealers. The active ingredient in the majority of medicated sealers is paraformaldehyde, which is usually accompanied by a corticosteroid. Figure 24 shows a medicolegal case where excess medicated sealer entered the inferior dental canal, causing permanent nerve damage with paraesthesia of the lip and soft tissues.

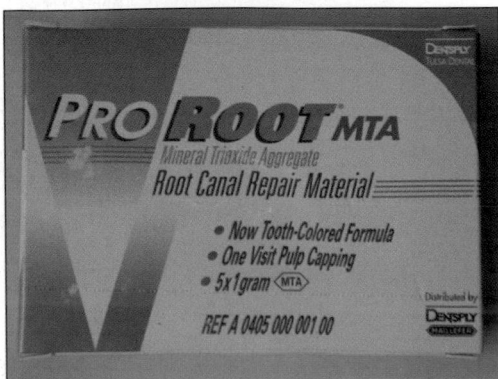

Fig. 25 Mineral Trioxide Aggregate is commercially available as Pro-Root.

Mineral trioxide aggregate

Mineral trioxide aggregate (Fig. 25) is a compound consisting of mineral oxides, (tricalcium silicate, tricalcium oxide, silicate oxide and traces of other mineral oxides), developed first by Mahmoud Torabinejad and co-workers at Loma Linda University.[10] Although originally developed as a root-end filling material during periradicular surgery, researchers across the world have reported positive results when the material is used for the repair of perforations, as a pulp capping agent, and to induce apical closure of immature roots. The superb sealing ability, marginal adaptation and biological compatibility of the material appear to make this material the sealant of choice for any communication between the root canal system and the external surface of the tooth. The material is continually being refined, and the latest product has some oxides removed to produce a white, rather than grey, powder. MTA is a difficult material to manipulate, having the consistency of wet sand. Methods of placement are described in Part 11.

Root canal filling instruments
Spreaders

Cold lateral compaction using gutta-percha requires either long-handled or finger spreaders (Fig. 26). These have a long, tapered shank with a sharp point. The instrument is used to compact gutta-percha laterally against the walls of the root canal and provide a space for the insertion of further gutta-percha points. There are several sizes available, and these are selected according to the canal size and the size of the gutta-percha point. The choice of long-handled spreaders or finger spreaders depends on personal preference. The advantage of finger spreaders is that less force can be used, and this reduces the risk of root fracture.

Heat carriers

The application of heat to the gutta-percha filling permits improved lateral and vertical compaction of the softened material. Ordinary hand and finger spreaders are not designed for this purpose, but the instruments illustrated in Figure 27 may be used. They are of various sizes, and have both a pointed tip for lateral spreading, and a flat tip for vertical compaction.

The instrument shown in Figure 28 is a System B, for the controlled and precise application of heat to the gutta-percha filling. Figure 29 shows an Obtura machine, used to deliver heated gutta-percha directly to the root canal. The use of these and other similar machines is described in Part 8.

Magnification

When asked why endodontics is a difficult subject, undergraduate and postgraduate students alike frequently reply that it is because they cannot see what they are doing. There is no doubt that magnification of the pulp chamber greatly assists in finding and accessing narrow canal orifices, and many practitioners now routinely use loupes, as seen in Figure 30. This one purchase has made huge improvements in the quality and ease of endodontic treatment by many practitioners. Indeed, the improved vision gained from the use of loupes improves all aspects of general dental practice, not just endodontics. The patient in the illustration is merely undergoing a routine examination.

However, specialist practitioners, and some generalists, are moving to the use of surgical microscopes, as seen in Figure 31 where it is being used by a relatively new member of staff in training, who was seeking, and found, a sclerosed canal in an upper incisor.

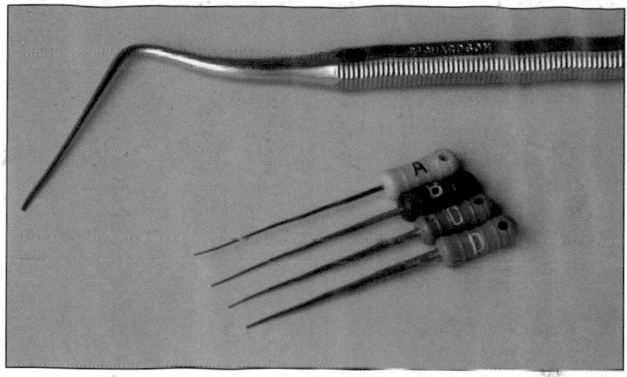

Fig. 26 Cold lateral compaction may be carried out with either finger spreaders or long-handled spreaders.

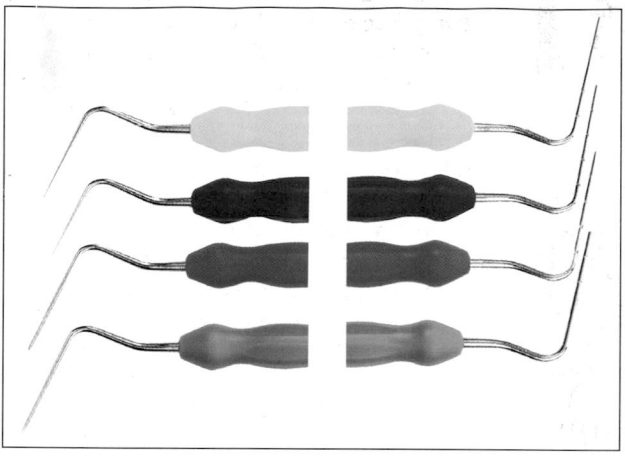

Fig. 27 Machtou heat carrier/pluggers for warm lateral and vertical compaction.

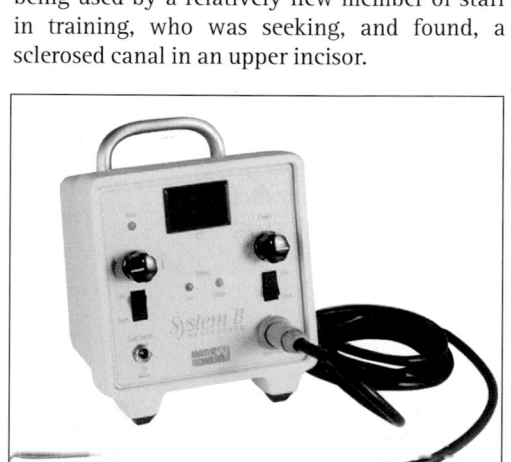

Fig. 28 The System B heat source for controlled warm gutta-percha techniques.

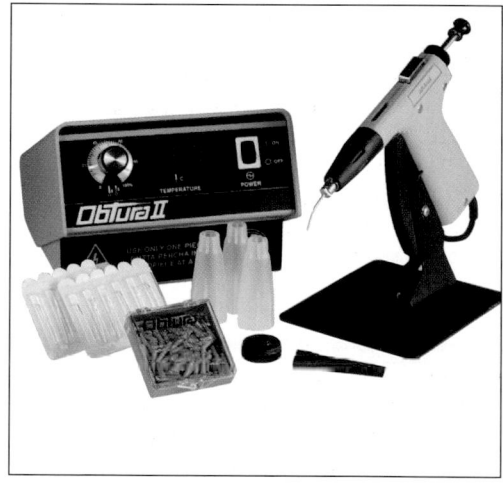

Fig. 29 The Obtura 11 system for injecting heat-softened gutta-percha into the root canal.

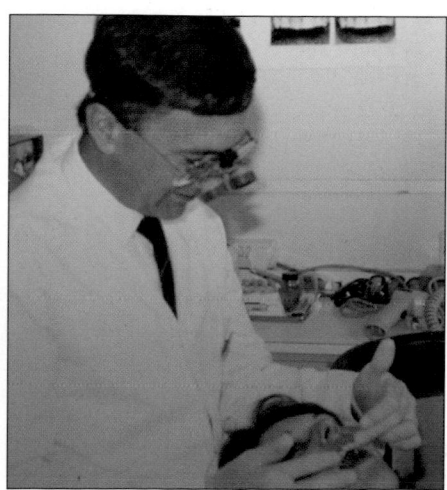

Fig. 30 The use of magnifying loupes is increasing in restorative dentistry.

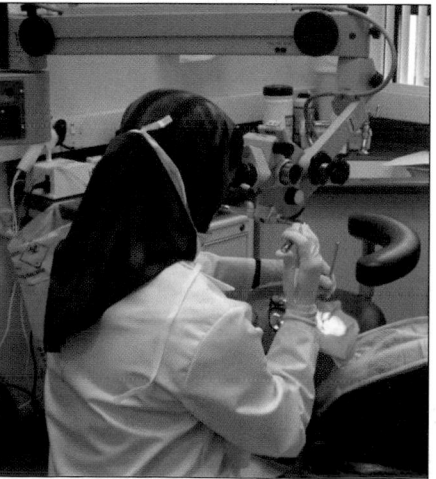

Fig. 31 A surgical microscope may be essential for some of today's intricate endodontic procedures.

1. National Radiographic Protection Board. *Guidance Notes for Dental Practitioners on the safe use of x-ray equipment.* 2001 Department of Health, London, UK.
2. Cameron J A. The synergistic relationship between ultrasound and sodium hypochlorite: a scanning electron microscope evaluation. *J Endod* 1987; 13: 541–545.
3. Byström A, Sundqvist G. Bacteriological evaluation of the effect of 0.5% sodium hypochlorite in endodontic therapy. *Oral Surgery, Oral Medicine, Oral Pathology* 1983; 55: 307–312.
4. Solovyeva A M, Dummer P M. Cleaning effectiveness of root canal irrigation with electrochemically activated anolyte and catholyte solutions: a pilot study. *Int Endod J* 2000: 33: 494–504.
5. Haffner C, Benz C, Folwaczny A, Mech A, Hickel R. High frequency current in endodontic therapy; an in-vitro study. *J Dent Res* 1999; 78: 117.
6. Ranta K, Haapasalo M, Ranta H. Monoinfection of root canals with Pseudomonas aeruginosa. *Endod Dent Traumatol* 1988; 4: 269–272.
7. Smith A J, Dickson M, Aitken J, Bagg J. Contaminated dental instruments. *Journal of Hospital Infection* 2002 (in press).
8. Lowe A H, Bagg J, Burke F J T, MacKenzie D, McHugh S. A study of blood contamination of Siqveland matrix bands. *BDJ* 2002; 192: 43–45.
9. Tronstad L, Barnett F, Flax M. Solubility and biocompatibility of calcium hydroxide-containing root canal sealers. *Endod Dent Traumatol* 1988; 4: 152–159.
10. Torabinejad M, Hong C U, McDonald F, Pitt Ford T R. Physical and chemical properties of a new root-end filling material. *J Endod* 1995; 21:349–353.

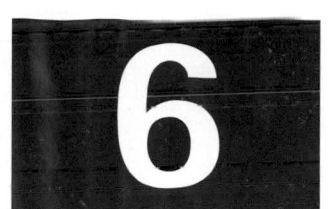
IN BRIEF
- Rubber dam is essential for effective isolation of the root canal and operating field from salivary bacteria, as well as protection of the airway.
- Only a very small number of rubber dam clamps are required for the efficient application of rubber dam, which must be supported by a well-trained dental nurse.
- Success in modern endodontic treatment may be dependant upon a well-designed access cavity to permit straight-line access to all the main root canals.

Rubber dam and access cavities

Rubber dam is easy to apply once the basic components and principles are understood. An efficient and well-trained dental nurse will greatly facilitate the application procedure. Although preparation of the access cavity may be commenced before rubber dam is applied to enable anatomical landmarks to be followed, the rubber dam should be placed as soon as possible with adequate protection against contamination of the access. The access cavity reflects the shape of the pulp chamber, modified by the angle of instrument approach.

RUBBER DAM

The use of a rubber dam is almost mandatory in modern endodontic practice for three reasons.

Firstly, it provides an aseptic operating field, isolating the tooth from oral and salivary contamination. It cannot be stressed enough that contamination of the root canal with saliva introduces new microorganisms to the root canal which may prolong treatment and reduce prognosis.

Secondly, rubber dam facilitates the use of the strong medicaments necessary to clean the root canal system.

Finally, it protects the patient from the inhalation or ingestion of endodontic instruments, as shown in Figure 1.

Practitioners may also be advised to develop their rubber dam skills for another reason. Research has shown[1] that rubber dam used during routine conservation procedures reduces aerosol contamination and cross-infection by up to 98.5%.

Research has also shown that patients do not dislike the use of rubber dam,[2] and the author has never had a single patient request its removal once the reasons for its use have been explained. It may be particularly helpful to explain to the patient that the rubber dam is necessary to isolate the operating area in exactly the same way as a surgical drape is essential for similar invasive medical procedures, where bacterial contamination may have a profound effect on the outcome. Indeed, refusal to accept a rubber dam may preclude the prescription of endodontic therapy. If an endodontic instrument is inhaled, a medicolegal allegation of negligence may be impossible to defend, even if the patient had appeared to accept the risk. A practitioner should never do anything to a patient which he or she knows to be wrong, and a patient may not sign away their rights in law.

With a little practice, an understanding of the basic principles, a well organized surgery and a well-trained dental nurse, a single tooth can be isolated in only a few seconds.

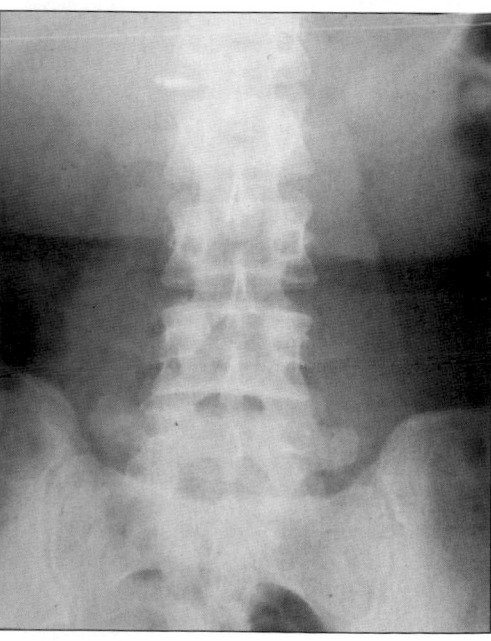

Fig. 1 An endodontic instrument has been inhaled due to a lack of airway protection.

Fig. 2 A modern single table rubber dam punch.

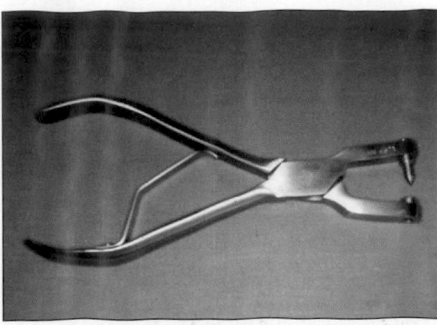

Fig. 3 For multiple isolation, the position of the holes to be punched may be marked by holding the rubber dam against the teeth.

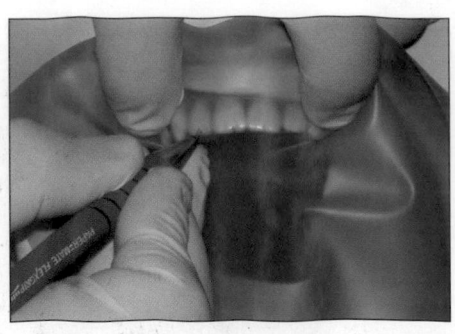

Rubber dam sheets

Most manufacturers supply rubber dam in three thicknesses or grades, for different applications. Depending upon the manufacturer, these will be designated either light, medium and heavy, or medium, heavy and extra-heavy. The thinnest of the three is more prone to splitting, and the heaviest more difficult to manipulate, which means that the most widely used is the middle grade. The sheets are presented in a variety of colours, some being impregnated with peppermint and other scents to disguise the smell of the rubber. The feel of rubber against the skin may be countered by simply placing a gauze underneath the dam.

A pack of latex free dam is also necessary for patients with latex allergies. This material appears slightly stiff at first but stretching the sheet a few times makes it easier to handle.

Rubber dam punch

Much of the equipment for rubber dam has been rationally modified. The revolving plate on the old punch was rarely used, as a single size hole will really fit all teeth. When the table was moved it frequently led to eccentric wear of the pin, which then did not cut a clean hole. The

defect in the cut may cause the dam to split when stretched out. The new rubber dam punches are single table (Fig. 2) and should always cut a clean hole. If they do not, they should be returned to the supplier.

Rubber dam stamp

This is another piece of equipment now largely superseded. For single tooth isolation, a hole punched 2 cm diagonally from the middle of the sheet gives universal dam. The hole is simply orientated to the quadrant under treatment. For multiple isolation, it is preferable to hold the dam against the teeth to be isolated, and mark the centre of each tooth with a pen, as shown in Figure 3. The holes will then be punched in accordance with the patient's dentition and not with an arbitrary stamp.

Rubber dam forceps

The rubber dam forceps are used to carry the clamp to the tooth. The most frequently reported problem with rubber dam is that when the clamp has been expanded and placed on the tooth, the forceps are stuck in the clamp and cannot be removed! This is because the grooves in the tips of the forceps are too deep. These should be modified with a stone or sandpaper disc so that they just engage the clamp, but slide off easily. Most forceps have a second groove slightly distant from the tip, which may be used to remove the rubber dam clamp without re-engaging the holes (Figs 4 and 5). There are several designs of forceps, and they may be employed with either an over-hand or under-hand grip – experimentation will reveal the most comfortable.

Fig. 4 The tips of the rubber dam forceps on the right have been modified for ease of use.

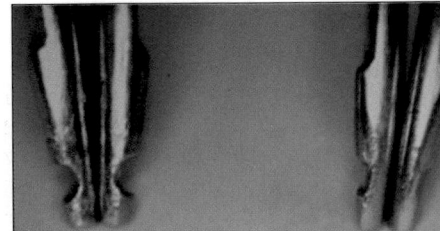

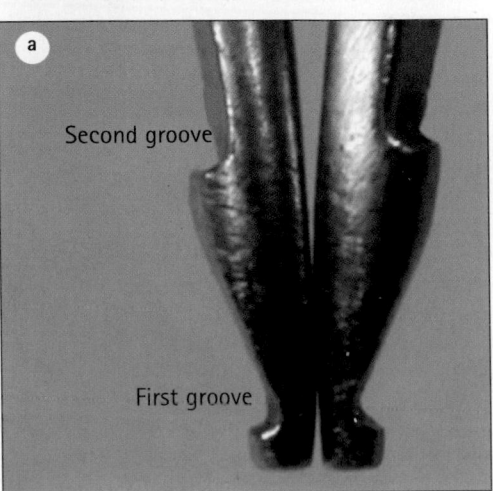

Second groove

First groove

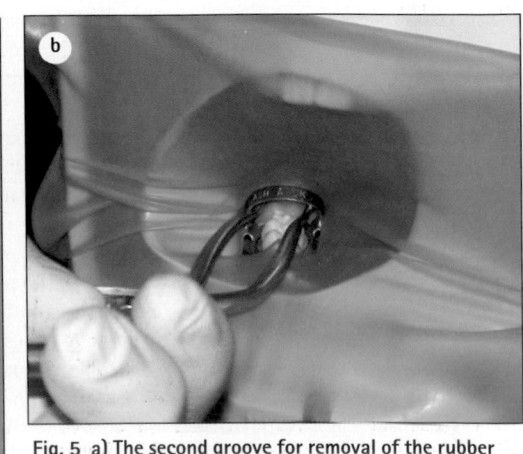

Fig. 5 a) The second groove for removal of the rubber dam clamp, as shown in b).

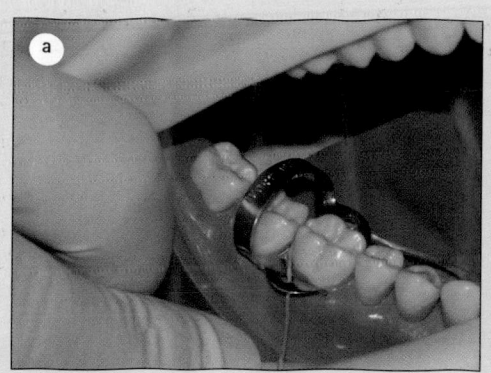

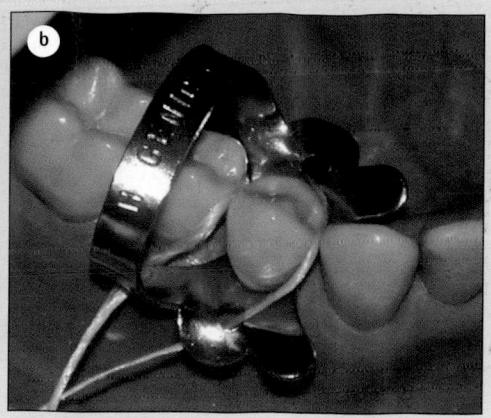

Fig. 6 Universal molar and premolar clamps, demonstrated on a phantom head. a) A wingless molar clamp (W8a).

b) A winged premolar clamp (1)

Rubber dam clamps

There is a vast range of shapes and sizes of rubber dam clamps, supposedly to suit every possible tooth and situation. In fact, this merely causes confusion, as an ill-fitting clamp may be quite unsatisfactory, and dislodge during treatment. When properly fitted, a clamp should have four-point contact with the tooth. If not, it will either rock back and forward or dislodge completely.

Clamps are described as being either 'active', where the jaws slope downwards and positively slide into cervical undercuts, or 'passive' when they tend to remain where placed. They may also be either winged or wingless, depending upon the chosen method of application.

The size 8A clamp is described by the manufacturers as a 'universal retentive molar clamp'.

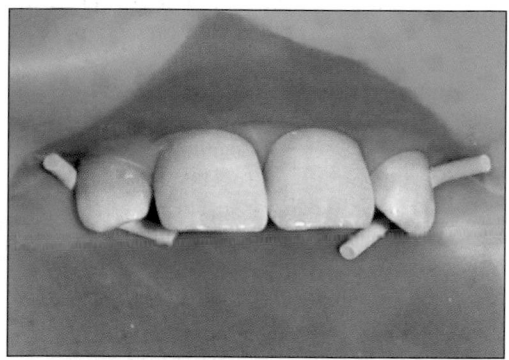

Fig. 7 Wedgets may be used in place of clamps for anterior teeth.

It is an active clamp, and fits every molar tooth, even when these are quite broken down. The author would suggest therefore that all the other designs merely confuse the issue, and until the operator is very experienced only this clamp is used for all molar teeth. Likewise, the size 1 fits virtually all premolars (Fig. 6). If passive clamps are preferred size 0 or 00 are suitable for premolars, although they will not be as retentive. Rather than place aggressive clamps on anterior teeth, it is usually kinder to use interproximal wedges, either pieces of rubber dam or a commercial product such as 'Wedgets' (Fig. 7). It is often easier to isolate several anterior teeth, giving a clear operating field.

Occasionally, a clamp may be dropped in the patient's mouth, or may fracture across the bow as seen in Figure 8, during application. All rubber dam clamps should be protected with a length of dental floss, about 50 cm, threaded through the holes on either side. It is not necessary for this to be wrapped around the clamp as was described in some early restorative textbooks. Indeed this should not be done since, once the clamp is in place above the rubber dam sheet and technically outside the mouth, the floss should be cut and withdrawn. If not it may act as a wick, drawing saliva into the operating field, or taking medicaments down into the mouth. Small voids around the dam may be sealed with a caulking agent such as Oraseal or Cavit (Fig. 9).

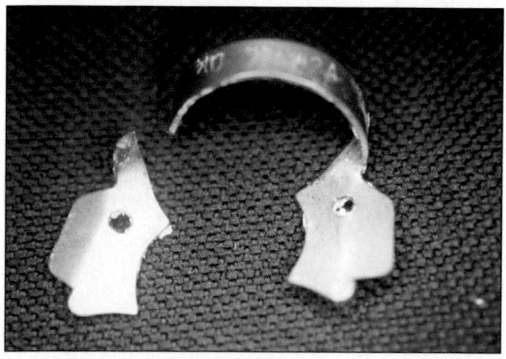

Fig. 8 Rubber dam clamps should always be protected with a length of dental floss in case they either fracture, as shown here, or are dropped in an unprotected mouth.

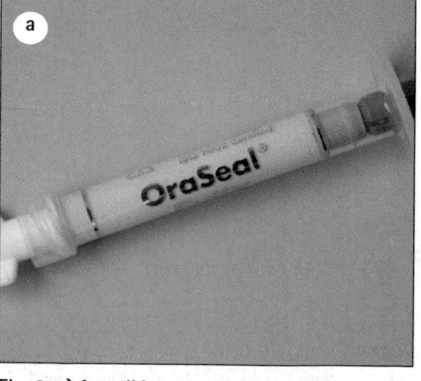

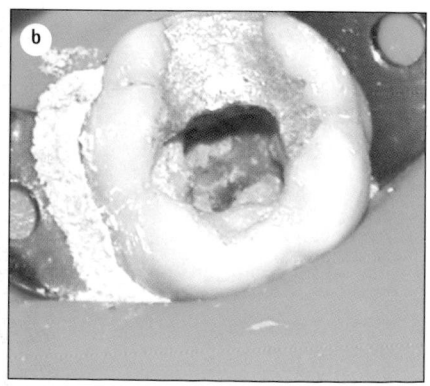

Fig. 9 a) A caulking agent which may be used to seal voids around the rubber dam that may allow salivary contamination, as shown in b).

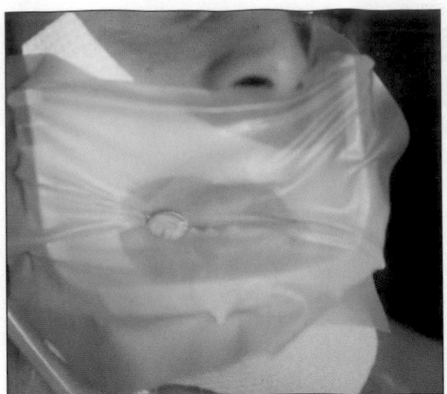

Fig. 10 The rubber dam frame may be easier to place beneath the rubber sheet.

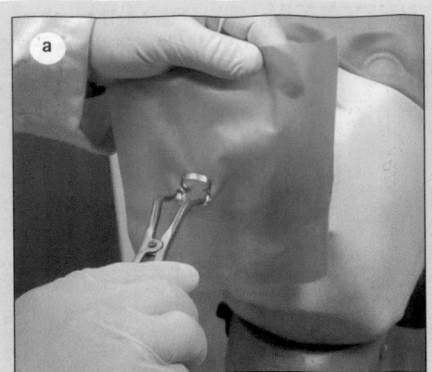
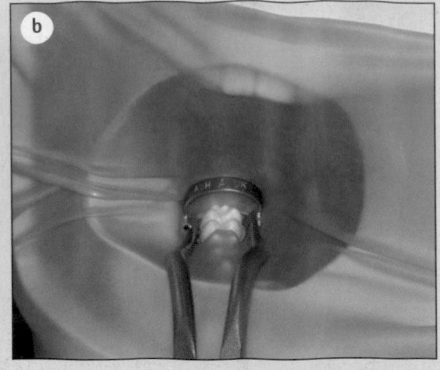

Fig. 11 The winged technique. The hole in the rubber sheet has been stretched over the wings of the clamp a), which is then fitted to the tooth b). The rubber is pushed off the wings, and the seal verified.

The rubber dam frame

The old Ash frame, with its 'butterfly' retainers, has largely been replaced by plastic or metal frames with sharp points or pins. It should be noted that the majority of these retentive points slope backwards, and the frames are designed to be placed under the rubber dam (Fig. 10). It seems to be much easier to place the frame beneath the dam and simply stretch the sheet over the points than the other way round. In addition, the tension in the sheet can be better controlled, particularly relevant when working in a situation where the clamp may be less retentive than normal.

For comfort, most patients appreciate a small piece of gauze placed between the rubber and their skin, and some practitioners place a prop (an old McKesson anaesthetic type) between the teeth on the non-working side to relieve the patient's muscle tension.

APPLICATION TECHNIQUES

A well-trained dental nurse and a well organized surgery, are essential for efficient application of the rubber dam. If a tray is prepared with ready punched sheets, and sterilized clamps already flossed, application can be performed in a matter of seconds.

There are three standard methods of application, described and illustrated here.

Winged technique

The appropriate winged clamp (8A for molars, 1 for premolars) is selected and flossed. The rubber dam is punched and aligned with the quadrant to be treated. The clamp is held in the forceps and retained with the ratchet. The hole in the rubber is stretched across the wings of the clamp, positioning the bow of the clamp towards the back of the arch. All this may be done by the dental nurse while the dentist is otherwise occupied, perhaps administering the local anaesthetic. The nurse then holds the top of the sheet to improve vision for the operator, who simply places the clamp onto the tooth to be treated (Fig. 11). A flat plastic instrument is then used to push the rubber off the wings, and the frame and gauze are applied. The floss may then be removed and the seal verified or adjusted as necessary.

Wingless technique

The appropriate wingless clamp (W8A for molars, W1 for premolars) is selected and flossed. The rubber dam is punched and aligned with the quadrant to be treated. The clamp, held in the forceps and retained with the ratchet, is placed securely on the tooth. One advantage of this method is that the opportunity now exists to verify the fit of the clamp before proceeding (Fig. 12). The rubber dam is now held in both hands, and the index fingers used to stretch out the punched hole, which is slipped over the bow

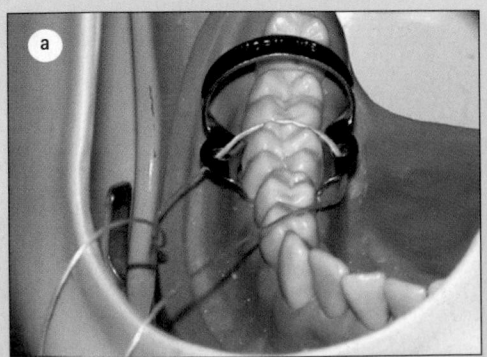
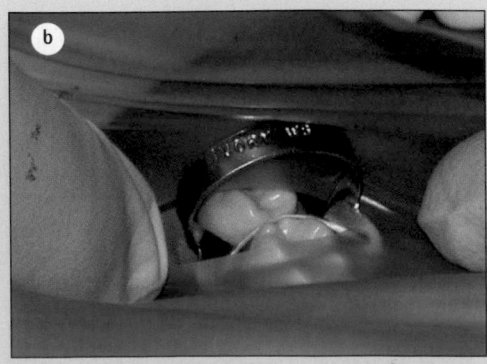

Fig. 12 The wingless technique. a) The flossed clamp has been placed on the tooth, and b) the rubber is stretched over the bow and pulled forward around the clamp.

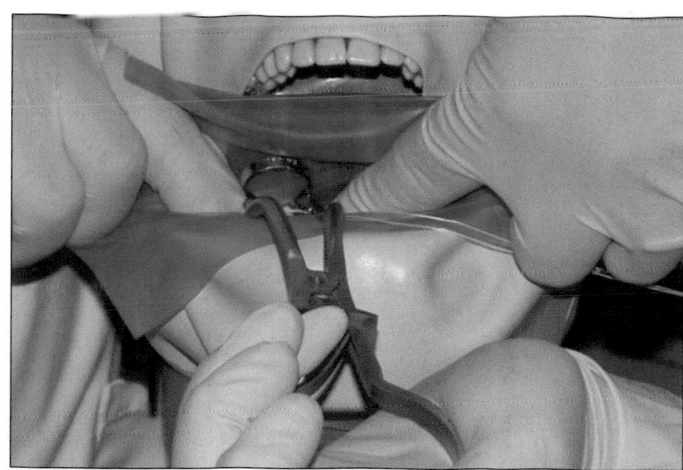

Fig. 13 The rubber first method. The operator is holding the sheet over the tooth whilst the assistant places the clamp to secure it in place.

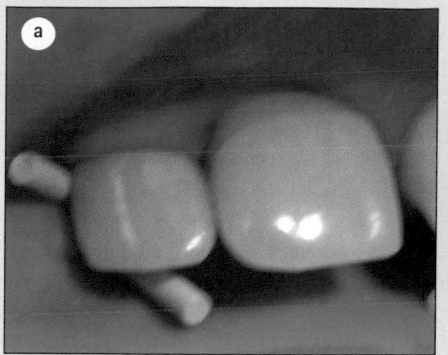
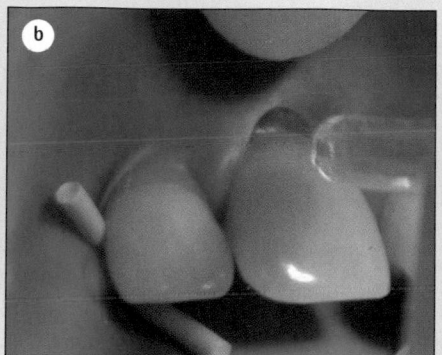
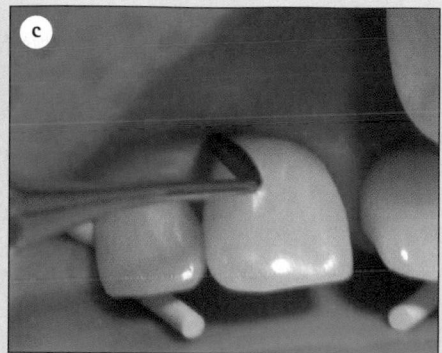

Fig. 14 a) The rubber dam is lying on the tooth surface and may allow leakage. It should be everted into the gingival crevice by

b) stretching the rubber away from the tooth and drying the mucosa with a stream of cold air, before

c) using a flat plastic instrument to tuck the rubber into the crevice.

of the clamp and pulled forward and down onto the tooth. Again, the nurse may hold the top of the sheet to improve vision for the operator. The frame and gauze are applied, the floss removed and the seal verified or adjusted as necessary.

Rubber first

The third method taught in some centres involves the dental nurse to a greater extent. The dentist stretches out the rubber and places the hole over the tooth in question, holding it down on each side with light finger pressure. At the same time the dental nurse picks up the flossed clamp in the forceps and places it over the tooth, retaining the dam in place (Fig. 13). Once again, the frame and gauze are applied, the floss removed and the seal verified or adjusted as necessary.

Anterior teeth

As stated previously, in a relatively intact arch it is easier to isolate several anterior teeth. Dental floss should be used first to verify that the contacts are clear and that the rubber dam will pass through. The rubber sheet is held against the teeth and the centre point marked of those teeth to be isolated. Holes are punched at these points, and the rubber dam is then applied to the teeth. Taking a leading edge of rubber through the contact – 'knifing through' – makes application relatively simple, or dental floss may be used to draw the rubber through a difficult contact. Once in place the selected wedges are applied.

Everting the margins

If the rubber dam is lying on the tooth surface it may allow leakage of saliva, a problem particularly when the dam has been applied during adhesive restorative procedures, but also with endodontics. The margin should be everted into the gingival crevice as shown in Figure 14. The operator stretches the rubber away from the tooth whilst the assistant directs a stream of cold air from the triple syringe onto the mucosa. With the use of a flat plastic instrument the margin of the rubber dam may be tucked into the gingival crevice, providing a tight seal.

Alternatively, some operators apply floss ligatures, as shown in Figure 15, using a flat plastic

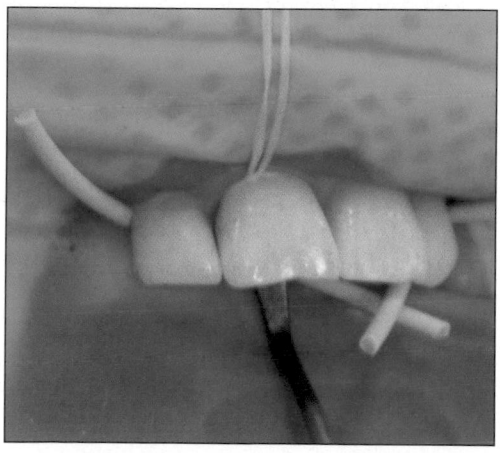

Fig. 15 Alternatively, floss ligatures may be used to hold the rubber dam in the gingival crevice. Ligatures will be applied to each tooth under treatment.

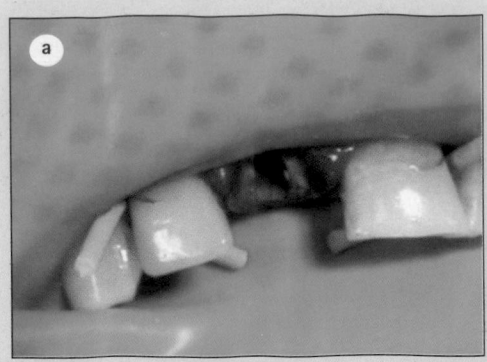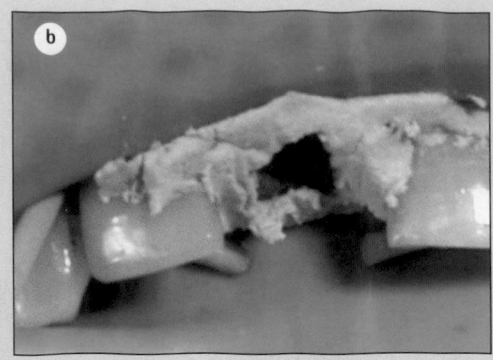

Fig. 16 a) A slot has been cut in the rubber dam to enable this root to be isolated. b) However, it is essential that a caulking material is applied to prevent salivary contamination.

to push the floss above the cingulum, and tying a knot securely on the labial aspect of the tooth.

DIFFICULT SITUATIONS
There are a few situations where the application of rubber dam may present difficulties, although the cautious clinician may consider whether root canal treatment is then either appropriate, or may be severely compromised.

The broken down tooth
The broken down tooth may be tackled in a variety of ways. Many molar teeth with large deficiencies may have rubber dam applied, providing the right clamp is used; the author recommends a W8a (see Fig. 2). With an appropriate length of floss as described earlier, the clamp is placed directly on to the tooth, so that there is a four-point contact between the jaws of clamp and the root. Once in position, the clamp is checked for stability by pressing on the bow. If firm, the rubber dam may be stretched over the clamp using the wingless technique described.

It is also feasible to build up the tooth before commencing root canal treatment using glass ionomer (for example, Vitremer). Alternatively, an orthodontic band may be cemented around the tooth. On occasion, a clamp may be fitted on to a broken down tooth, but only if the gingival tissue encroaching on to the margin is first removed with electrosurgery or a surgical blade.

As part of the restorative treatment, periodontal crown lengthening, or orthodontic extrusion, may be indicated. These procedures should be carried out prior to commencing the root canal treatment.

Bridges
Bridges do not present a problem with the application of rubber dam. A suitable winged clamp is fitted onto the abutment tooth and the dam stretched over the clamp. If there are any small gaps, these can be sealed with a caulking material such as Oraseal or Cavit.

When root treating teeth acting as bridge abutments a careful check should always be made that the bridge is not loose. If a bridge has become debonded it must be removed. This should be carried out before any attempt is made to root-treat one of the abutment teeth.

Split dam
Occasionally, a broken down tooth may be isolated using a slit cut between the holes made for the two adjacent teeth, as shown in Figure 16. It is essential that the caulking material illustrated in Figure 9 is applied to prevent leakage and contamination.

Finally, if an operator decides to proceed with root canal treatment without the use of rubber dam, each hand file must be protected with either floss tied around the handle or an appropriate safety device. The excess saliva must be controlled with cotton wool rolls and aspiration, and great care must be taken with medicaments. It would be advisable to inform the patient of the risks involved, and the reduced prognosis for the treatment if salivary contamination of the root canal occurs.

ACCESS
Access cavity preparation
There is an old cliché that 'Access is Success'. Unlike other aspects of dentistry, root canal treatment is carried out with little visual guidance; therefore, the difficulties that are likely to be encountered need to be considered. An assessment of the following features can be made after visual examination of the tooth, and study of a pre-operative periapical radiograph taken with a paralleling technique:

- The external morphology of the tooth.
- The architecture of the tooth's root canal system.
- The number of canals present.
- The length, direction and degree of curvature of each canal.
- Any branching or division of the main canals.
- The relationship of the canal orifice(s) to the pulp chamber and to the external surface of the tooth.
- The presence and location of any lateral canals.
- The position and size of the pulp chamber and its distance from the occlusal surface.
- Any related pathology.

Before commencement of root canal treatment, the tooth must be prepared as follows:

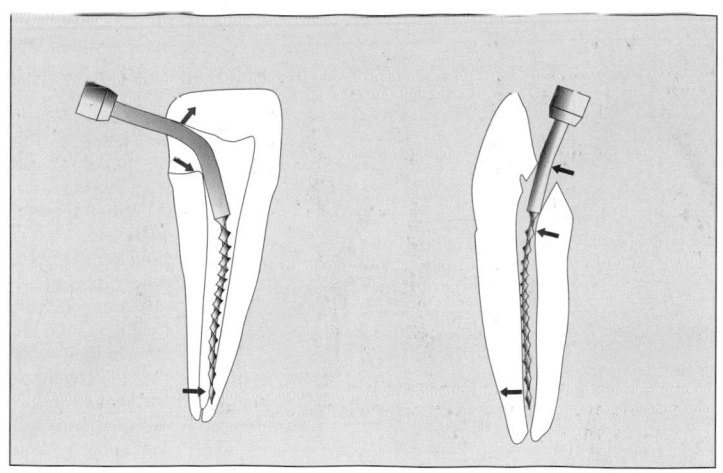

Fig. 17 This diagram illustrates the importance of straight line access and correctly designed access cavities. If root canal treatment were to be carried out through a Class III cavity, as shown on the left, the file would be deflected and the canal would be transported. However, if the access cavity is cut incorrectly in the palatal surface, not giving straight line access, the same deflection and damage will occur.

- All caries and any defective restorations should be removed and made good. The tooth should be protected against fracture during treatment.
- The tooth should be capable of isolation.
- The periodontal status should be sound, or capable of resolution.

It may be prudent to commence access cavity preparation before isolating the tooth with rubber dam in order that the anatomical landmarks, tooth inclination and other helpful features are not lost. It is, of course, crucial that the root canal does not become contaminated during either access preparation or canal instrumentation, and the tooth should be isolated in an aseptic field as soon as possible.

If there is a danger of fracture of the coronal tooth structure, the cuspal height should be reduced to prevent this. If the loss of coronal tissue is extensive, there may be a need to provisionally restore the tooth with a temporary crown, copper ring or an orthodontic band. It is, however, not always necessary to restore the tooth before carrying out endodontic procedures. Provided the tooth will anchor a rubber dam, the canals can be isolated from the oral cavity and a temporary seal can be placed over the canals, this will be sufficient.

The objectives of access cavity preparation are to:

- Remove the entire roof of the pulp chamber so that the pulp chamber can be debrided.
- Enable the root canals to be located and instrumented by providing direct straight line access to the apical third of the root canals, as illustrated in Figure 6.17. Note that the initial access cavity may have to be modified during treatment to achieve this.
- Enable a temporary seal to be placed securely in order to withstand any displacing forces.
- Conserve as much sound tooth tissue as possible and as is consistent with treatment objectives.

The subsequent restoration of the tooth should always be considered first. If the tooth is not heavily restored then only the amount of coronal tissue sufficient for the successful completion of the root canal treatment should be removed. However, if the tooth is already compromised and will require some form of cuspal coverage restoration, an onlay or a crown, then it may be practical to reduce the cusp height, particularly mesiobuccally in molars, to enable better visualization of the pulp chamber. If access to the back of the mouth is difficult, it is again reasonable to consider reducing the marginal ridge of the tooth concerned to achieve this (Fig. 18), or perhaps gain access through the mesiobuccal wall. Unless the root treatment is successful, any further restoration to the tooth will be put at risk.

Before beginning the access cavity preparation, it is wise to check the depth of the preparation by aligning the bur and handpiece against the radiograph, in order to note the position and depth of the roof of the pulp chamber in relation to the length of the bur in the handpiece (Fig. 19). Particular note should be made of the position of the largest pulp horn.

The stages of access cavity preparation may be summarized as follows:

1. The initial entry is made with a tungsten carbide or diamond bur in a turbine handpiece and the outline form completed as required. The bur is advanced towards the pulp horns until the roof of the pulp chamber is just penetrated. (Note particularly that in a molar tooth the bur approaches the tooth from the mesial and from the buccal. Thus the access

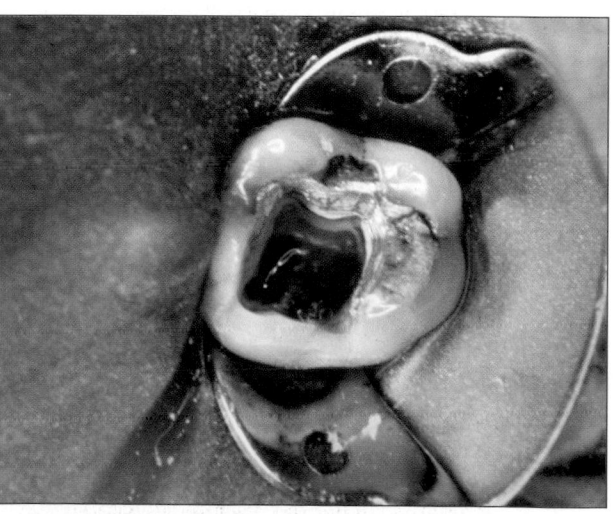

Fig. 18 Reducing the mesial marginal ridge may be necessary to permit clear visualization of the pulp chamber.

Fig. 19 The pre-operative radiograph should be examined carefully for suitable landmarks before commencing the access cavity. Here, the depth of penetration of the bur is being estimated.

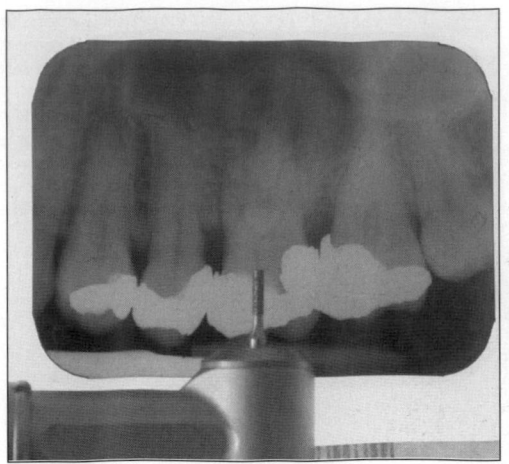

Fig. 19 The pre-operative radiograph should be examined carefully for suitable landmarks before commencing the access cavity. Here, the depth of penetration of the bur is being estimated.

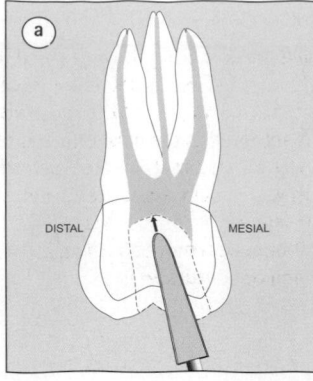

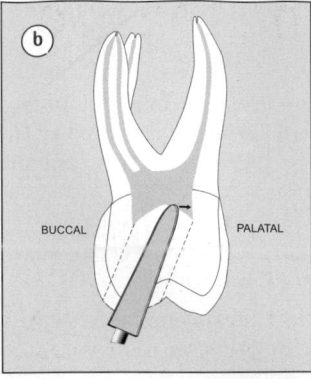

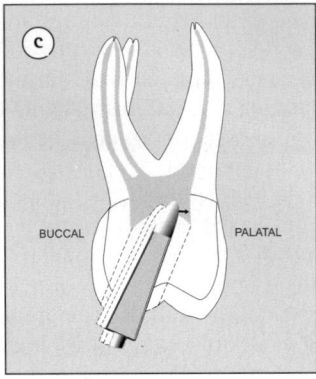

Fig. 20 These diagrams illustrate how, in a molar tooth, the bur approaches the pulp chamber from the mesial (a) and from the buccal (b). When the roof of the pulp chamber has been penetrated, a safe-tipped bur (c) should be used to remove the roof of the pulp chamber and shape the walls without damaging the floor and canal orifices.

cavity is cut in the mesiobuccal segment of the occlusal surface.)

2. At this point, the rubber dam should be applied if it is not already in place.

3. The removal of the entire roof of the pulp chamber, and the tapering of the walls, is now carried out with a safe-tipped endodontic access bur, as described in Part 5. (Stages 1 and 3 are illustrated in the diagrams in Fig. 20.)

4. The walls of the pulp chamber may now be gently flared out towards the occlusal surface. The end result should be a gentle funnel-shape, with the larger diameter at the occlusal surface. The safe tip of the bur will be felt passively following the contours of the floor of the pulp chamber.

5. Any remaining pulp tissue and debris is cleared with an excavator from the floor of the pulp chamber and the canal orifices.

6. The access cavity should be flushed with a solution of sodium hypochlorite to remove any residual debris.

7. The canal orifices may be located with a DG 16 endodontic probe. Any alteration to the access cavity outline form may now be undertaken to ensure a direct line of approach to the canal orifices. Any sclerotic or secondary dentine surrounding the canal orifices may be removed with a CT4 tip in a piezo-electronic ultrasonic machine.

8. Once the canal orifices have been identified, the preparation of the coronal part of the root canals should be commenced. Depending upon the operator's preferred technique, either Gates–Glidden burs or nickel-titanium orifice shapers, should be employed. Copious irrigation is necessary, together with the use of a canal lubricant containing EDTA. These techniques are described in Part 7.

9. An access cavity must be seen as dynamic, with modifications being made as treatment progresses to permit the straightest possible access of instruments.

10. It can only be repeated that access is success. If the access cavity is not large enough to permit easy and thorough shaping and cleaning of the entire root canal system, the root canal treatment may be compromised and the tooth lost.

1. Marshall K. Dental workspace contamination and the role of rubber dam. *CPD Dentistry* 2001; 2: 48-50.
2. Gergely E J. Rubber dam acceptance. *BDJ* 1989; 167: 249-252.

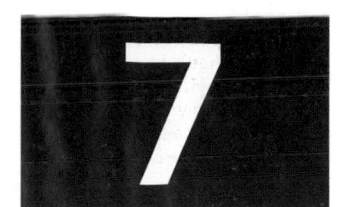

IN BRIEF

● Modern techniques for preparing the root canal involve a crown-down approach to more efficiently remove infected debris and to improve access for irrigants.
● The balanced-force technique, with a 60° clockwise turn followed by a balanced anti-clockwise cutting motion, is accepted as the most efficient method of file manipulation, (except that when using Hand GT files the motions are reversed).
● Copious irrigation with an appropriate antiseptic material is essential to clean the root canal system following shaping of the main canals.
● The smear layer should be removed with an EDTA solution before placing an intervisit dressing, or carrying out obturation.

Preparing the root canal

Research into root canal preparation has led to significant changes in instrumentation techniques. Hand files should be manipulated by the balanced-force technique. Recent designs of endodontic instruments have variable tapers giving improved shaping ability. Nickel Titanium rotary instruments will rapidly and safely open the main root canals creating deep space to permit full permeation of irrigant solutions. Practitioners considering changing their endodontic technique are advised to attend hands-on practical courses to gain competence before using these in clinical practice.

Success in endodontic treatment depends almost completely on how well the root canal is shaped and cleaned. This part will cover the principles of root canal preparation, irrigation, root length determination, intracanal medication, and temporary fillings.

There have been more developments in recent years in this aspect of endodontic practice than any other. New instruments have been developed, employing different metals and different engineering philosophies. There has been a significant move away from the ISO standard 2% taper instrumentation.

Two root canal preparation techniques using hand instruments will be described in detail, as these are the standard techniques currently taught in most dental schools, and are considered to be the most efficient and suitable for clinical dental practice. Details are also given of the use of engine-driven rotary instruments.

PRINCIPLES AND RECENT DEVELOPMENTS OF ROOT CANAL PREPARATION

The principles of root canal preparation are to remove all organic debris and microorganisms from the root canal system, and to shape the walls of the root canal to facilitate that cleaning and the subsequent obturation of the entire root canal space. However, a tooth root rarely contains a single simple root canal. Accessory canals, lateral canals, fins, anastomoses between canals, and an apical delta all contribute to the root canal system, as shown in Part 1. The majority of these anatomical features are not accessible to instrumentation. An irrigant solution must be used which can be flushed through this system, will destroy the microorganisms and preferably dissolve organic debris at the same time. Thus the current concept of root canal preparation is not *cleaning and shaping*, but *shaping and cleaning*. The main root canals should be rapidly and efficiently shaped with instruments to permit thorough and extended cleaning of the entire pulpal system with the irrigant solution.

Once shaped and cleaned, the root canal system is obturated to prevent further ingress of microorganisms, both apically and coronally, and to entomb any remaining microorganisms to prevent their proliferation. Currently, the root canal filling material of choice is gutta-percha, which requires a gradual, even, funnel-shaped preparation with the widest part coronally and the narrowest part at the apical constriction, normally approximately 1.0 mm short of the root apex (Fig. 1). Wide, relatively straight canals are simple to prepare, but fine, curved canals can present considerable difficulties. In the past, a number of techniques have been described, all of which have been designed to produce a tapered preparation.

DEVELOPMENT OF PREPARATION TECHNIQUES

In order to fully understand the current techniques for canal preparation, it would be beneficial to look briefly at previous methods, and the associated problems which led to further development. Interestingly, in 1933 a paper was published in the dental literature recommending the use of maggots to consume and remove the necrotic

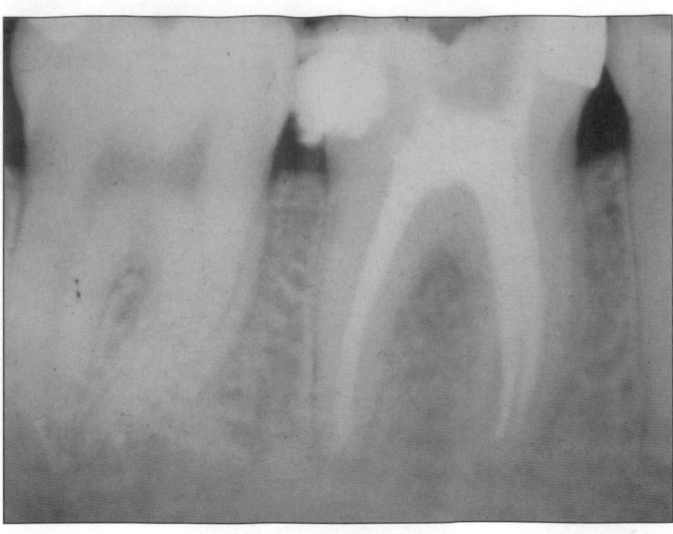

Fig. 1 The shape of the prepared root canal should be a gradual, even taper, with the widest part coronally and the narrowest part 1.0 mm from the root apex.

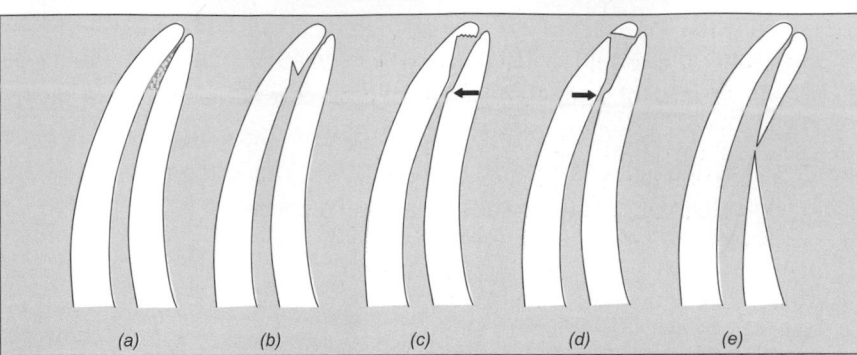

(a) (b) (c) (d) (e)

Fig. 2 Procedural errors in the preparation of curved canals. a) Dentine debris and pulp remnants packed into the apical part of the canal resulting in loss of working length. This may be avoided by recapitulation with fine files and copious irrigation. b) Ledging due either to not precurving the instrument, or forcing it into the canal. c) Apical zip caused by rotating the file excessively. d) Perforation due either to persistent filing with too large an instrument, or continual zipping. Note the narrower part of the canal in c) and d) is termed an elbow. This makes obturation of the root canal very difficult in the widened apical area. e) Strip perforation caused by overpreparing and straightening the curved canal.

tissue in the root canal, replacing them every 3 days. It soon became apparent that more objective and controllable techniques were required!

The standardized system

This technique was used for many years and required each instrument, file or reamer, to be placed to the full working length. The canal was enlarged until clean white dentine shavings were seen on the apical few millimetres of the instrument. The filing was continued for a further two or three sizes, to complete the preparation. This method was satisfactory in straight canals, but was quite unsuitable for curved canals. As the instrument sizes increase, they become less flexible and led to iatrogenic errors in curved root canals. Common problems encountered were ledging, zipping, elbow formation, perforation and loss of working length owing to compaction of dentine debris (Fig. 2).

The stepback technique

The stepback technique was devised to overcome the problem of the curved root canal and has been described by Mullaney.[1] The apical region is first enlarged using files to a final master apical file size 25 or 30; each successively larger instrument is then inserted 1.0 mm less into the canal so that a taper is formed. In between placing each larger instrument, the master apical file is inserted to the working length to clear any debris collecting in the apical part of the canal; this is referred to as recapitulation.

The stepback technique helped to overcome the procedural errors of the standardized technique in slight to moderately curved canals, but in the more severely curved root canals problems still exist. There are three ways in which some of the problems of the curved root canal may be overcome, by using:

- A special filing technique.
- A file with a modified non-cutting tip.
- More flexible instruments.

Stepdown technique

This method, although not the term stepdown, was first suggested by Schilder in 1974, and the technique was described in detail by Goerig et al.[2] It has been followed by other, similar techniques such as the double flared[3] and the crown-down pressureless.[4] The principle of these techniques is that the coronal aspect of the root canal is widened and cleaned before the apical part (Fig. 3). The obvious advantages of these methods over the stepback are as follows.

- It permits straighter access to the apical region of the root canal.
- It eliminates dentinal interferences found in the coronal two-thirds of the canal, allowing apical instrumentation to be accomplished quickly and efficiently.
- The bulk of the pulp tissue debris and microorganisms are removed before apical instrumentation is commenced, which greatly reduces the risk of extruding material through the apical foramen and causing periapical inflammation. This should reduce the incidence of after-pain following preparation of the root canal.
- The enlargement of the coronal portion first has several benefits. It allows better penetration of the irrigating solution to the entire root canal system and forms a reservoir of irrigant which is more readily replenished in the canal system. It also reduces the risk of compacting debris apically which may block the canal.

The stepdown technique is now the most widely used technique for canal preparation, and will be described later in this part.

INSTRUMENT MANIPULATION

In addition to the method of approach to the root canal, there have been numerous techniques for the manipulation of endodontic shaping instruments.

Watchwinding and circumferential filing

Watchwinding, or a continuous back and forth rotation with slight apical pressure, rapidly advances a fine file down a root canal. Each

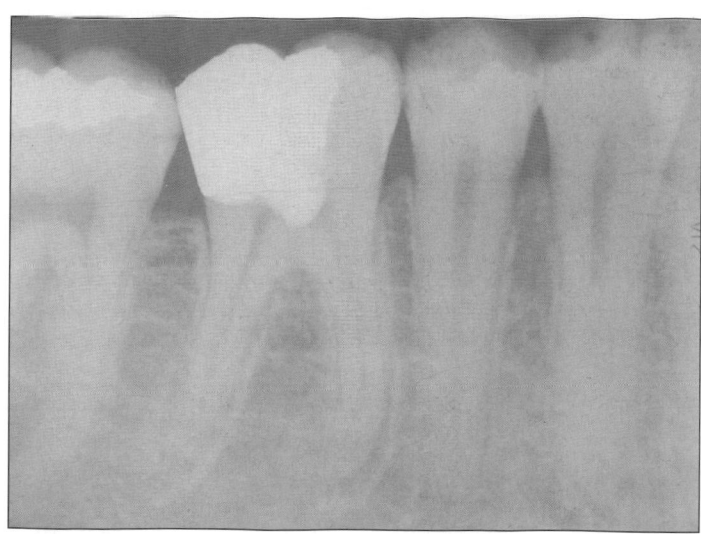

Fig. 3 The root canal in this tooth contains necrotic infected debris. The objective in endodontics is to remove the debris without extruding any through the apical foramen. It makes good sense to use a technique which cleans the coronal part first and then the apical portion.

slight turn engages the flutes of the file in the canal wall and removes dentine. Only fine files should be advanced to the apex in this way as there is a danger of compacting pulpal debris ahead of the file. If such a blockage occurs it can be extremely difficult to remove.

Once the file has reached the desired length, a push-pull filing action was used, moving the file circumferentially around the canal walls. When using K-type files an attempt was made to file on the outstroke only, again to reduce the apical compaction of debris. Hedstroem files were more efficient for circumferential filing, although these should not be used when watchwinding. Research into canal preparation found two distinct problems with circumferential filing.

The first was a tendency to preferentially file the inside wall of a curved canal. The technique of anticurvature filing was put forward by Abou-Rass *et al.*[5] Anticurvature filing involves filing predominantly away from the inner curve of a root to reduce the risk of a strip perforation. The mesiobuccal roots of maxillary molars and the mesial roots of mandibular molars are the teeth most frequently at risk. The method is used only in canals with a moderate-to-severe curve.

The second finding was that once the file engaged in the coronal part of the root canal, the apical flutes tended not to cut dentine but remain passive. The majority of the filing occurred coronally, which tended to leave underprepared canals which were not fully cleaned.

The balanced force technique

The balanced force technique, first described by Roane *et al.*,[6] is now the most widely taught technique for manipulating handfiles. It is particularly good when negotiating the curved root canal. The technique requires flexible files with non-cutting tips. The file is inserted into the canal until slight resistance is felt and then rotated 60° clockwise to engage the flutes into the dentine. If a greater movement is made, iatrogenic problems can quickly arise. Using light apical finger pressure to hold the file at exactly the same depth in the canal, the file is

now rotated through 360° in an anticlockwise direction. The first 60° of this turn cuts off the dentine engaged in the flutes of the file, and the remainder of the movement picks up this dentine in the flutes of the file prior to the next cycle. The amount of apical pressure required to rotate the file anticlockwise is just sufficient to prevent it from winding out of the canal. Watching the rubber stop in relation to the tooth assists in keeping the file steady with no in or out movement.

If the file is engaged too far into dentine with the first clockwise movement, ie if the turn is greater than 60°, excessive force is applied to the file during the cutting phase, and the file may fracture. The balanced force cycle of movement should be made no more than three times before the file is withdrawn to be cleaned, ideally by pressing it into a sterile sponge. The root canal system should be irrigated copiously before the file is reintroduced. Using this method, curved canals may be prepared to the full working length without producing apical transportation.

Ultrasonic technique

Ultrasound has been used to activate specially designed endodontic files. Ultrasound consists of acoustic waves which have a frequency higher than can be perceived by a human ear. The acoustic energy is transmitted to the root canal instrument, which oscillates at 20–40,000 cycles per second, depending on which unit is used. The superior cleaning effect is achieved by acoustic streaming of the irrigant and not, as originally thought, by cavitation.[7] Irrigation with sodium hypochlorite is necessary,[8] although some of the ultrasonic units are not designed to accept sodium hypochlorite through the system and, if water is used, they will be less efficient in their cleansing effect. Even when units designed to take sodium hypochlorite are used, daily maintenance must be carried out to prevent damage, particularly to metals, because the irrigant is corrosive.

The irrigant passes down the shank of the instrument and into the root canal, producing a continuous and most efficient system. Acoustic

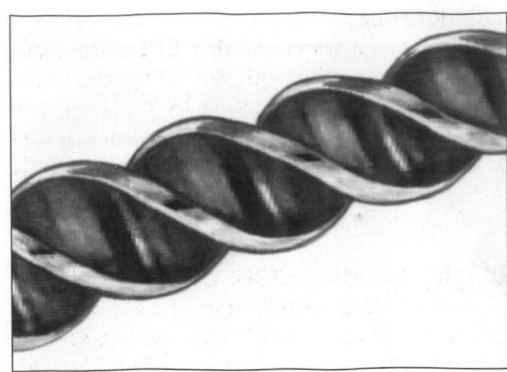

Fig. 4 A diagram of a nickel–titanium rotary file showing the concept of radial lands.

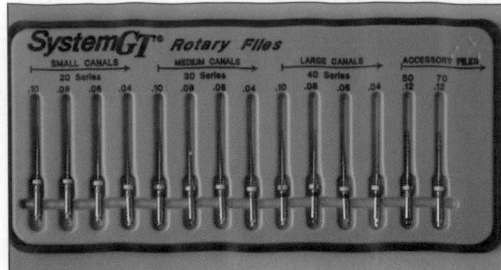

Fig. 5 One modern system of nickel–titanium rotary instruments — the System GT.

streaming is produced by the rapid file oscillations in the irrigant within the root canal. With more recent developments, ultrasonic machines are now largely used for their efficient irrigation properties rather than for canal shaping.

Automated devices

There have been many automated handpieces on the market over the years which claim to make the preparation of root canals quicker and more efficient. Although different designs and mechanical actions have been tried, they have all suffered from the inherent difficulties referred to earlier, caused by rotating or twisting conventional stainless steel instruments, such as zipping, perforation, canal transportation and broken instruments.

Nickel–titanium

However, the development of nickel-titanium alloys has revolutionized automated root canal preparation. The remarkable ability of these alloys to alter their crystalline state gives instruments manufactured from nickel-titanium profound flexibility. Mechanized instruments can withstand the distortions caused by repeated rotation in curved canals without causing preparation errors. Most of these instruments have design features such as radial lands (Fig. 4) to keep the instrument centred in the canal, and a non-cutting tip to guide the instrument down the canal. New designs are constantly appearing, (Fig. 5) and the clinician should ensure that considerable experience with whichever system is chosen has been obtained on extracted teeth, before the instruments are introduced into clinical patient treatment.

A controlled high-torque, low-speed motor is required for efficient use of the instruments. Most manufacturers of endodontic instruments produce such a motor, and their complexity may vary from that illustrated in Part 5, Figure 12, to that shown here in Figure 6. It must be emphasized that these nickel-titanium instruments do have a limited life, and will fracture in time after a large number of rotations. Slow (150–250 rpm) rotation does not impede their efficiency but extends their life. However, it is recommended that the instruments should be discarded after a certain number of cases as described by the

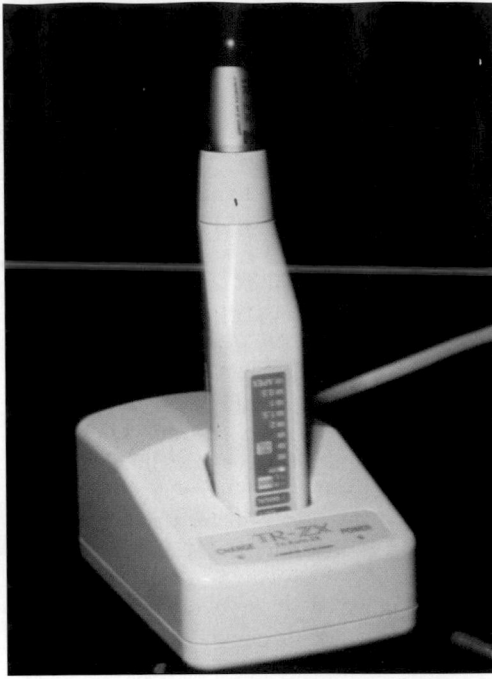

Fig. 6 A 'state-of-the-art' endodontic motor, being a rechargeable slow-speed, high-torque handpiece encompassing an apex locator and associated facilities.

manufacturer, and more frequently if an instrument has been used to negotiate difficult curved canals. The files should also be removed from the canal and cleaned frequently. Although debris is moved coronally it tends to compact in the file flutes, and if these become occluded the instrument will fracture. The separated part will engage in the root canal and may prove extremely difficult to remove.

IRRIGATION
Sodium hypochlorite

The importance of effective irrigation in root canal preparation cannot be overemphasized. A maxim in endodontics states that it is what you take out of a root canal that is important, not what you put in. Sodium hypochlorite is considered the most effective irrigant, as it is bactericidal, dissolves organic debris and is only a mild irritant. It must be clearly understood that almost any irrigant solution will cause an inflammatory reaction in the periapical tissues if it is expressed under pressure.[9] Great care must be taken to follow the irrigation regime described below.

There is considerable debate about the recommended or optimum concentration of sodium hypochlorite. Ordinary domestic bleach, such as that purchased from any supermarket, has approximately 5% available chlorine. This may be used neat, or may be diluted with purified water BP up to 5 times. Greater dilutions do not affect the antibacterial properties, but diminish the tissue dissolution property. Diluted solutions must therefore remain in the root canal for longer. Warming the irrigant makes it even more effective.[10] There are other commercially available sodium hypochlorite products, but it must be emphasized that there should be no other additives, particularly sodium chloride.

During preparation, the root canal should be kept wet, with copious irrigation used after each instrument. The irrigant in the canal is only replaced to the depth of insertion of the needle. The needle must remain loose in the canal while the irrigant is being injected, to prevent the solution being expelled under pressure into the periapical tissues. To obtain total replacement of irrigant solution in the root canal, the smallest needle available (30-gauge) should be placed at the apical foramen. Obviously, this is a most hazardous procedure and it is suggested that the irrigation needle is only inserted to a maximum depth of 2.0 mm short of the working length. A file may then be worked in the apical 2.0 mm, to stir and withdraw the dentine debris further into the canal, so that it can be flushed away. There are several differently designed irrigation needle tips, but in the author's opinion these are of little importance compared with the diameter of the needle. Whatever the tip design, unless the needle can penetrate loosely to the correct depth in the root canal, irrigation, however copious, will not remove dentinal debris.

Chlorhexidine

As referred to in Part 5, some practitioners have concerns about the use of sodium hypochlorite and prefer to use a solution of chlorhexidine. Whilst this has a similar antibacterial spectrum, it does not have the ability to dissolve organic debris and may not clean the entire root canal system as effectively. However, chlorhexidine does exhibit substantivity (adherence to dentine) and there is some evidence to suggest that it may be a more appropriate irrigant for retreatment of failed orthograde cases where sodium hypochlorite was the original irrigant.

Ethylene–diamene tetracetic acid (EDTA) solution

Endodontic instrumentation creates a smear layer on the root canal walls, particularly when using nickel-titanium rotary instruments. This smear layer occludes the dentinal tubules, and may protect microorganisms from the effects of the sodium hypochlorite irrigation. Flushing the canal with EDTA solution (Fig. 7) periodically during instrumentation removes the smear layer, and enables more effective cleansing. The final irrigation should always be with sodium hypochlorite.

LUBRICATION

Proprietory pastes containing EDTA are available, in combination with various agents, which greatly help instrumentation by chelating and softening the dentine. If a small portion is dispensed near to the file storage system, a little may be picked up on the tip of each new file as it is selected (Fig. 8).

DETERMINATION OF ROOT CANAL LENGTH

The exact apical termination of the root canal preparation has always been a subject of contention. The pedantic answer is that the root canal should be prepared to that point where the 'inside' of the tooth becomes the 'outside'. Some authors suggest this is the apical constriction, some the cemento-dentinal junction, some suggest that the apical foramen should be enlarged, some suggest that the preparation be taken to an arbitrary point 1 mm from the radiographic apex. As described in Part 4, the apical anatomy may be complex, and the term apical delta may be more appropriate. This author considers that the preparation should be taken as close as possible to the cemento-dentinal junction, and that wherever possible the foramen of the major canal should be kept patent. (This technique is described later.) The other minor canals forming the apical delta will only be cleaned by antibacterial irrigation flushing through the entire canal system.

An estimate of the root length is made from the pre-operative radiograph taken with a parallel technique. However, confirmation of the actual working length is not carried out until the coronal preparation of the canal has been completed, as this may straighten a curved canal which would change a measurement that had been taken too early. Most operators now confirm the actual working length when the crown-down preparation has progressed to within 3 or 4 mm of the estimated working length. There are three accepted methods for this determination.

Working length radiograph

A file is placed carefully in the canal until it is within approximately 2.0 mm of the overall length. Before insertion the file should be pre-curved to the shape of the canal and gently manoeuvred into position, if necessary using a watchwinding technique and slight apical pressure. For accurate reading of the radiograph a size 15 file is usually necessary. A silicone stop

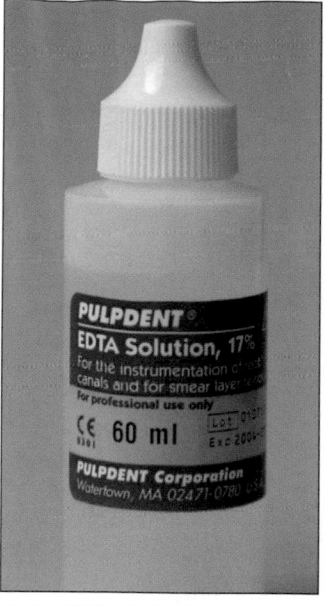

Fig. 7 EDTA solution for final flushing of the canal system.

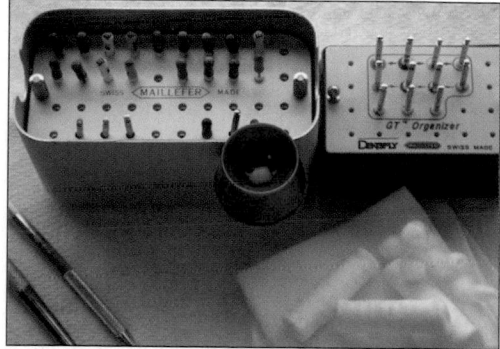

Fig. 8 EDTA paste should be placed near the files and picked up on each instrument before use.

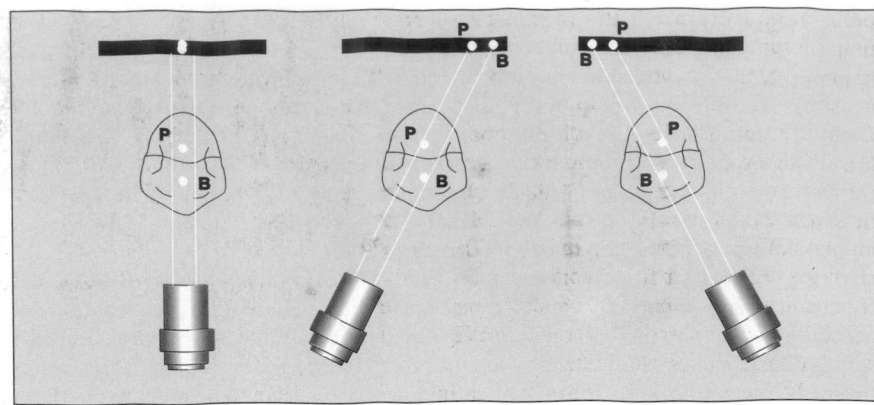

Fig. 9 The buccal object rule. When the x-ray cone is moved to the mesial and directed distally, the buccal canal will appear the most distal on the radiograph.

on the instrument shank is positioned against a reference point on the tooth, and both the length and the reference point should be noted in the records. When taking diagnostic radiographs, use should be made of the 'buccal object rule', where there are two or more canals present in the root (Figs 9 and 10). A second way of achieving the same result is to place a Hedstroem file in one canal and a K-file in the other, as the difference between the two is clear on the radiograph. The working length is calculated by measuring directly on the radiograph from the tip of the instrument to 1.0 mm short of the radiographic apex. It is only possible to estimate this arbitrary position using this technique.

Electronic apex locators

Electronic apex locators (seen in Part 5, Fig. 15) may be used as an alternative to a working-length radiograph, assuming that a pre-operative film has been examined to obtain an estimated figure. These machines are capable of accurate measurement, and will give the location of the apical foramen. Apex locators are essential when a patient elects to have a minimum number of further radiographs taken. Many practitioners now use them routinely, particularly when the outline of the canal on the pre-operative film is indistinct or the canal curves towards or away from the radiograph beam. Modern apex locators work using different frequencies, determining the ratio between the different electric potentials proportional to each impedance. There is no longer any need to

dry the canal before use as they work in the presence of electrolytes. There is a distinct learning curve with their use, but it is usually apparent whether or not the measurement is in accordance with the original radiographic estimated working length. Errors may occur if there is a large coronal restoration or metallic crown causing a short circuit; if there is an open apex with a large periradicular lesion, or if there is a perforation. These are usually apparent and further measures should be taken.

In use, a file is inserted into the root canal and an electrical contact is made with the shank of the instrument. The device has a second electrode, which is placed in contact with the patient's oral mucosa. A digital display or audible signal shows when the tip of the instrument reaches the apical foramen. There is no doubt that modern apex locators can be even more accurate in length determination than a radiograph.[11,12]

Tactile sensation

An experienced clinician, armed with an accurate pre-operative parallel radiograph, can often feel the apical constriction with a fine instrument. If tactile sensation is in accord with the estimated length, further confirmation may not be necessary.

PREPARATION OF THE ROOT CANAL

Two techniques will be presented in detail, one using conventional hand instrumentation and one using nickel-titanium hand Files of Greater Taper. The stepdown technique has been modified slightly from the original description by Goerig.[2] The use of nickel-titanium rotary instruments is presented in general terms only. As discussed earlier, there is a rapid development of these instruments, and the instructions and guidance of the manufacturers of the specific instruments chosen by the clinician should always be adhered to. It is strongly recommended that appropriate hands-on training is undertaken, practising the technique on a large number of extracted teeth before taking the new procedures to a patient.

STEPDOWN TECHNIQUE WITH CONVENTIONAL 2% TAPER INSTRUMENTS

A pre-operative radiograph is taken, rubber dam placed and an access cavity prepared. The canal

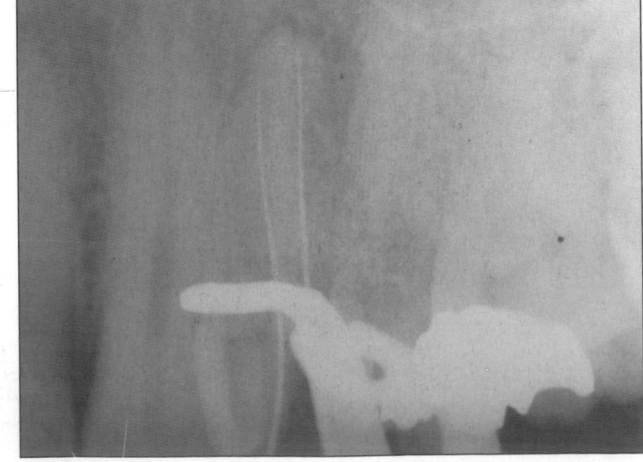

Fig. 10 The diagnostic radiograph was taken from the mesial with the x-ray cone pointing distally. The buccal canal is therefore the distal one on the radiograph.

preparation is divided into two parts: i) coronal preparation, which permits radicular access for ii) apical instrumentation.

Coronal preparation or radicular access

First, the pulp chamber is copiously irrigated with sodium hypochlorite. Gates–Glidden burs are next introduced into the canal, directed apically and laterally away from the furcation. The larger sizes are introduced first, working sequentially further down the canal with smaller sizes. Some canals will accept a size 6 bur, but normally a size 4 would be used first, followed by a size 3. Each bur will penetrate 2–3 mm further than the previous one. EDTA paste should be used with each bur, and the canal should be irrigated between each entry. Eventually, in a relatively straight canal, the No. 2 bur is inserted 10–12 mm into the canal from the occlusal reference point. In a curved canal the pre-operative radiograph should be checked for the maximum straight line penetration of the bur.

Gates–Glidden burs should be rotated with constant medium drill speed from the time they enter the canal until removed. Gates–Glidden burs must not be taken into a curve, or they will almost certainly fracture. If the shank of a bur does break, it usually does so near the handpiece head and may be retrieved easily from the tooth, as seen in Figure 11. However, if the head does become separated from the shank within the canal, removal may be extremely difficult.[13]

The bur may be flexed against the canal wall slightly on withdrawal to ensure that the natural shape of the canal is maintained. Thus a round canal will remain round, but an oval canal will be prepared to a smooth oval funnel. A wide oval or 'figure-of-eight' shape may need preparing at both extremities to produce a wide flare. Instrumentation with the stepdown technique in the radicular access is accomplished using only light pressure directed apically and away from the furcation, or perforation may result.

An alternative to Gates–Glidden burs is the use of standard flexible K-type files with safe tips, used with the balanced force technique. Following initial widening of the mouth of the canal only with a Gates–Glidden bur, the largest hand file which will enter the canal is selected and worked apically, using EDTA paste as a lubricant. Once penetration proves difficult the file should not be forced further, or fracture may result. The next size smaller file is selected, and sequentially smaller files used until the coronal preparation is complete.

Apical preparation

The coronal flaring already carried out makes access to the apical portion of the root easier, as there are no dentinal obstructions and access is more direct. Thus, once the coronal preparation is complete, flexible K-type files with safe tips may be used sequentially with the balanced force technique previously described. A size appropriate to the particular canal and the final size Gates–Glidden drill is selected, perhaps a

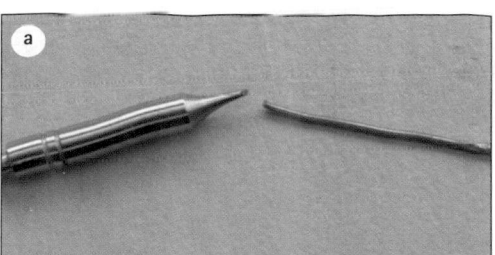
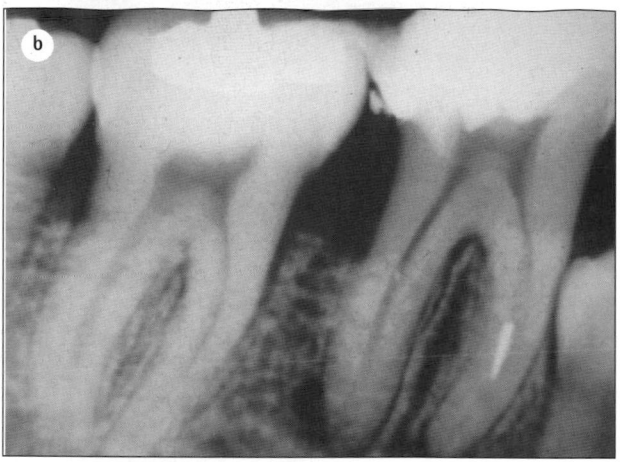

Fig. 11 A Gates–Glidden bur which fractured during use in the root canal, showing the normal point of separation, permitting removal with Steiglitz forceps. However, b) shows that this is not always the case.

size 60, the tip dipped into a canal lubricant, and the instrument worked slightly further into the canal. Sequentially smaller files are selected until the canal is prepared to 3–4 mm short of the estimated working length. Now the actual working length must be confirmed by one of the methods described earlier, radiograph or apex locator. Once the working length has been confirmed, the apical preparation can be completed. In narrow or sclerosed canals the operator may prefer to take a small 08, 10 and 15 files to working length before commencing any canal preparation. The prepared canal then acts as guidance for the larger sizes. This procedure is illustrated diagrammatically in Figure 12.

Stepback technique

Following the preparation of the coronal part of the root canal, the apical preparation may also be carried out using the stepback technique. Starting with the size 15 file at the working

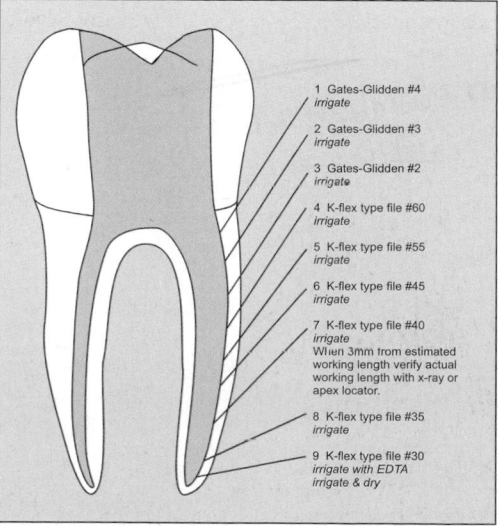

1 Gates-Glidden #4
irrigate

2 Gates-Glidden #3
irrigate

3 Gates-Glidden #2
irrigate

4 K-flex type file #60
irrigate

5 K-flex type file #55
irrigate

6 K-flex type file #45
irrigate

7 K-flex type file #40
irrigate
When 3mm from estimated working length verify actual working length with x-ray or apex locator.

8 K-flex type file #35
irrigate

9 K-flex type file #30
irrigate with EDTA
irrigate & dry

Fig. 12 A diagrammatic illustration of the sequence of instruments in a conventional 2% taper hand file canal preparation.

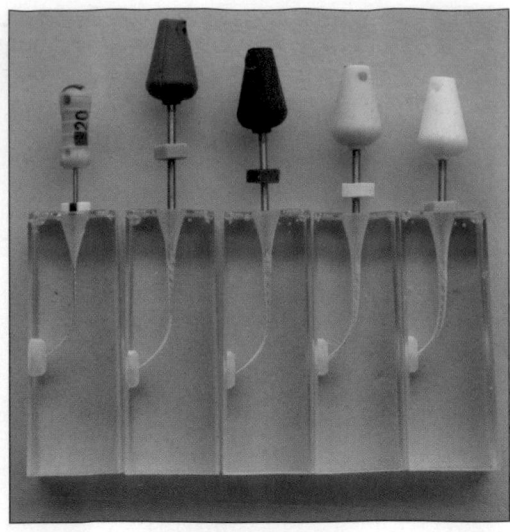

Fig. 13 An illustration of the steps involved in the preparation of a simulated root canal with Hand Files of Greater Taper.

length, and progressing to sizes 20 and 25, an apical stop is made. Copious irrigation and reca-pitulation with fine files will prevent build-up of canal debris. The master apical file will usually be no greater than 25 or 30. The apical portion of the canal is now tapered by stepping back. A file one size larger than the master apical file is worked with balanced force to 1.0 mm short of the working length. Each successively larger file

size is inserted 1.0 mm less than the previous size until the radicular access preparation is reached. In between each larger file selection the master apical file is inserted to full working length (recapitulation) and irrigation is used to remove all the debris.

STEPDOWN TECHNIQUE WITH HAND FILES OF GREATER TAPER

The stepdown technique may be modified with the use of this range of files described by Buchanan _ _ _.[14] The balanced force tech-nique is used as described previously, except that these instruments are used in the opposite rota-tion to conventional files. It was considered that the crucial part of the balanced force technique is the cutting cycle. Right-handed clinicians (repre-senting some 90% of the work-force) can make this movement more easily in a clockwise direc-tion than anticlockwise. Thus the initial move-ment to engage the dentine _with these files only_ is a 60° turn _anticlockwise_, and the balanced force cutting motion is 360° _clockwise_.

Following access to and irrigation of the pulp chamber the canal must first be gently explored to length with conventional 2% taper hand files. A gentle watchwinding technique is used with size 08, 10 and 15 files. The tip of the Greater Taper File then acts as a pathfinder rather than as a preparation file.

Using EDTA lubrication paste, the largest file with a blue handle and a taper of 12%, is used first to gain coronal access. When resistance is met the instrument is not forced further apically, but the red handled 10% taper file is used to penetrate further. The yellow handled 8% taper and white handled 6% taper follow in sequence, until the canal is prepared to working length.

The technique is varied according to the clini-cal situation. In a wide, straight canal, only a sin-gle 12% taper file may be required. In a narrow, curved canal, the clinician may only use the smaller files, alternating them repeatedly to create space for further apical penetration. Before attempting to instrument narrow, curved canals it is again always advisable to use conventional 2% taper instruments from size 08 through to size 20. The tip of the Greater Taper file then acts as a pathfinder, dentine removal occurring at the side of the instrument, not the tip.

Once a smooth-tapered canal has been pre-pared, the clinician may consider it necessary in some cases to enlarge the apical constriction slightly with conventional hand files.

The technique is summarized in Table 1, and shown in Figure 13.

NICKEL–TITANIUM ROTARY TECHNIQUE

The development and design of these instru-ments has been referred to earlier, and should be referred to in conjunction with this description of technique. Each manufacturer of these instru-ments produces a protocol for use for their own specific product. As it would not be appropriate to describe any single manufacturer's technique

Table 1 Root canal preparation using GT hand files

Aceess and coronal preparation

- Access – Remove roof of pulp chamber and locate canal orifices with the use of safe ended access Bur and DG16. Ensure straight line access to the canal orifice.
- Irrigate pulp chamber with sodium hypochlorite
- Estimate working length from pre-operative radiograph.
- Using a gentle watchwinding technique, and EDTA chelating agent/lubricant (File Eze/Glyde), advance a #08, #10, #15 and #20 K-type file to about 3 mm short of the estimated working length.
- If desired, with irrigation with NaOCl and with the use of the lubricant, open up the canal orifice using Orifice Shaper 4 & 3 crown down for approximately 3 or 4 mm. Orifice Shapers should be rotated at 250 rpm and used with a light pecking motion, keeping the instrument rotating within the canal at all times (Gates-Glidden drills can also be used for this procedure).

Mid–canal preparation

- Continue irrigation with NaOCl and the use of lubricant. Insert the #12 (BLUE) GT hand file within the canal and using a reverse balanced force action (60° turn anticlockwise followed by clockwise 180° turn with apical pressure – the 'balanced force') progress the file until resistance is felt and no further advancement of the file is possible. Do not use excessive force, and remove and clean the file after every three cycles.
- In the same manner insert the #10 (RED) GT hand file, repeating the procedure to penetrate further down the canal
- Either repeat the process with the #08 (YELLOW) hand file, or if approximately 3 mm from the estimated working length, proceed to:

Apical preparation

- Establish working length using electronic apex locator or with a diagnostic radiograph.
- Negotiate canal to full working length advancing #15 and #20 K-type files with watchwinding or balanced force motion.

Apical shaping

- Check canal patency using #15 K-type file with copious irrigation of NaOCl and use the #08 (YELLOW) GT hand file looking for resistance.
- Check canal patency before introducing the #06 (WHITE) GT hand file, this file should progress to full working length.
- Apical gauging can be checked or further enlarged with the use of K-type files.
- Continue irrigation with NaOCl for a total preparation time of 30 minutes, followed by final rinse of EDTA solution.

The above procedural protocol may have to be adapted taking into account the apical constriction, working length, apical curvature and general canal anatomy.

here, the description which follows must therefore be generic. The basic concepts are the same whatever the instrument chosen. The technique for use is crown-down, with copious irrigation. Indeed, these instruments conform totally to the stated objectives in modern root canal therapy, shaping the canal rapidly and efficiently so that thorough cleaning of the root canal system can be carried out with appropriate irrigants. The files must be used in a slow-speed, controlled torque motor, or they are prone to fracture.

Coronal preparation or radicular access

Nickel-titanium instruments cannot easily be precurved, and require straight line access to the root canal orifice. The use of ultrasonic tips to refine the access cavity has already been described. Nickel-titanium 'orifice shapers' have replaced Gates-Glidden drills, and may be used sequentially from the largest to the smallest sizes. These remain centred in the canal and will flare the canal walls to approximately halfway down the canal. Their use may be restricted in narrow or curved canals. They are used with a very light apical pressure, often described as the 'pencil-lead' pressure, ie that which would break the lead when using a propelling pencil. Each instrument should be used for no more than 5–10 seconds at a time before removing from the canal, cleaning, irrigating and adding lubricant.

Apical preparation

Once the coronal preparation is completed, the canal should be explored to full working length using fine hand files and the balanced force technique. The working length should be confirmed, and the canal enlarged to a size 15 or 20. If this is not done, the rotary instrument will have to cut at its tip, rather than along its length, which may lead to jamming and fracture. Each time a file is removed from a canal after use the position of the dentine debris in the flutes should be inspected. The instruments should cut along their entire length. If debris is only seen at the tip, the instrument may be excessively stressed, which may lead to fracture. The apical part of the canal may now be prepared with sequentially smaller instruments, stepping down the canal with each smaller size. It may be necessary to return to a larger size during preparation (recapitulation) to create more space for the smaller instruments.

Summary of technique

- Motor set at slow speed recommended for instrument, usually 150–250 rpm.
- Use each instrument for only 5–10 seconds.
- Light apical pressure, using either a gentle 'planing' pressure, or a slight 'pecking' motion depending upon the instrument design.
- Use EDTA lubricant with each instrument.
- Copious irrigation with sodium hypochlorite between instruments.
- Step down in sequence from the largest to the smallest. (NB This will depend upon which system is being used. If variable taper files

have been selected, as in Fig. 5, then a 10% taper file will be used until resistance is felt, moving to an 8%, 6% and 4% until any of these reaches working length, depending upon the canal size. Alternatively, if a single taper, variable tip system has been selected, the largest tip size will be used first, reducing sizes as the canal is negotiated until, once again, one instrument reaches working length.)

FURTHER READING

It must be stressed that the techniques described are generic, and that hands-on practice is essential, following the specific manufacturer's protocol until competence is achieved. The various instruments and techniques are described, compared and contrasted, in numerous publications, for example.[15-18] The prudent clinician would be advised to refer to the endodontic literature before embarking on new purchases and clinical practice. A useful series of clinical articles was presented by Buchanan.[19]

PATENCY FILING

Research has shown that most canal preparation techniques lead to the extrusion of debris through the apical foramen. This is removed by the normal body defence systems, although a certain amount of inflammation will result. Concern has been expressed by some authorities that such debris may remain in the apical constriction, and may contribute to failure, particularly if it harbours microorganisms.[20] The technique of patency filing involves passively inserting a small file, size 08 or 10, 2 mm beyond the established working length. No attempt is made to instrument the foramen, merely to keep it open or patent by deliberately extruding the debris into the periradicular tissues.

The literature on patency filing is at present quite equivocal. No research workers have been able to show either a decrease or an increase in post-operative symptoms or case prognosis. The technique remains subjective and subject to the operator's personal philosophy.

INTRACANAL MEDICATION
Calcium hydroxide

There is almost universal agreement that when an intervisit dressing is required, calcium hydroxide is the material of choice, and this is discussed in Part 9. There is far less agreement as to whether such dressings are indicated. Single-visit endodontics — the shaping, cleaning and obturation of the root canals in one appointment — remains controversial. Most endodontists would agree that when the tooth under treatment is not infected, for example when performing elective endodontics or treating large exposures of vital pulps, completing treatment in a single visit is advisable. However, Sjögren et al. showed a significant increase in prognosis when infected root canals were dressed with calcium hydroxide for one week before obturation.[21] Gutmann has suggested that this effect was only apparent because their research employed 1%

Fig. 14 A fine tipped plastic canula may be used to deliver medicaments deep into the root canal. Its size may be compared to the standard 28-gauge irrigating needle.

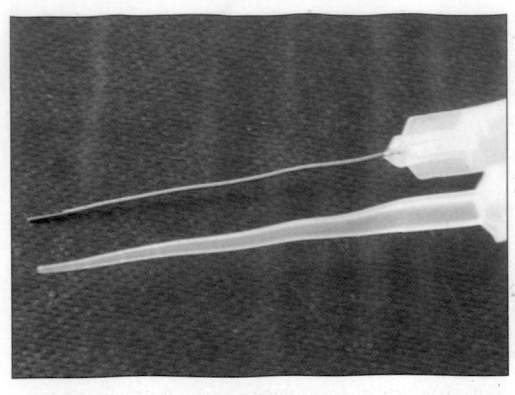

sodium hypochlorite, whereas the use of a full strength solution would preclude the need for such a dressing.[22] The wise practitioner would consider which approach best suits his or her style of practice.

Calcium hydroxide is applied with a spiral paste filler (noting the caution given at Part 5, Fig. 20), or a fine-tipped syringe may be used as seen in Figure 14. Care should always be taken not to extrude the material beyond the apical constriction. If this happens, inflammation may result which could take several days to subside. Calcium hydroxide containing points are available from which it is postulated that ions will dissociate into the fluid in the root canal, and which may be better controlled in apical length. However, research supporting this has not yet been reported in the endodontic literature.

A recent addition to the range of intracanal dressing available is the mixture Vitapex, shown at Figure 15. As well as calcium hydroxide, the material contains iodoform. It may be indicated for deep-seated infections of the root canal, such as the upper canine, shown in Part 2, Figure 1, which had resulted in an extra-oral sinus beneath the patient's eye. This closed and the tooth healed following one week's dressing. Extreme care is needed to ensure that this viscous dressing has been fully removed from the canal walls before obturation.

Steroids

Steroids are readily obtainable in the form of tri-amcinalone (Ledermix paste). The use of the paste for dressing an inflamed vital pulp prior to commencing root canal therapy is discussed in Part 3. Some authorities recommend the use of the paste as an intervisit medicament paste when severe periradicular inflammation is present. It is suggested that it may be wiped on the canal wall using a file or paper point which is then withdrawn; a small amount is then placed

on a pledget of cotton wool and sealed into the pulp chamber between appointments. The author prefers to mix the paste with a calcium hydroxide preparation, adding a little sterile water or local anaesthetic to make the mixture slightly more fluid. The canals may then be completely filled with this mixture prior to placing a temporary coronal seal.

Of course, no intracanal medicament yet exists that will sterilize the root canal, and the importance of biomechanical preparation cannot be stressed too strongly.

TEMPORARY RESTORATIVE MATERIALS

If endodontic treatment cannot be completed in one visit, it is essential that a temporary restorative material is used as an inter-appointment dressing that will not permit access to bacteria or oral fluids. Even when the root canal treatment has been completed, a well-sealed temporary restoration is necessary prior to the placement of a permanent restoration. The material should prevent contamination of the root canal system and must be sufficiently strong to withstand the forces of mastication.

Two different temporary materials are recommended. Of the many proprietary materials, Cavit has been shown to provide the best seal.[23] Cavit provides a good seal, is simple to apply and quick to set. On the other hand, it lacks strength and will not stand up to masticatory forces. It should be confined to single surface fillings for periods not exceeding a week. However, the shape of an endodontic access cavity is not retentive, and all such materials will either leak or be lost entirely in time. Any ingress of microorganisms may reinfect a prepared canal, and the time saved by using a rapid technique may be severely lost if such leakage occurs. Thus the use of a glass-ionomer cement should be considered. It is adhesive, antibacterial, stands up well to forces of mastication and is more stable than other materials.

It is a useful routine, with an inter-appointment dressing, to place a sterile pledget of cotton wool in the pulp chamber, followed by a layer of gutta-percha. The temporary restorative material is then placed over the gutta-percha (Fig. 16). At the next visit, a high-speed bur may be used to remove the temporary restoration without any danger of filling material lodging in the canal entrances or blocking the canals. The gutta-percha provides a base for the restorative material and prevents the bur becoming caught in the cotton wool when the temporary filling is removed.

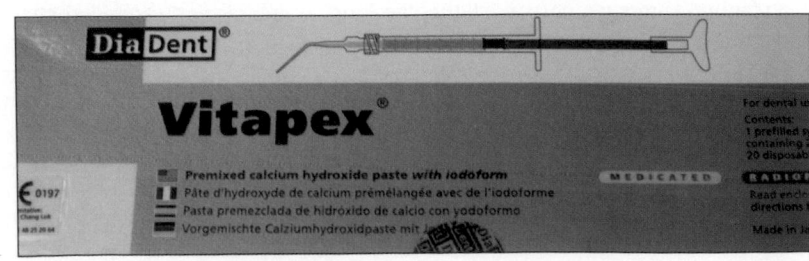

Fig. 15 Vitapex intracanal dressing.

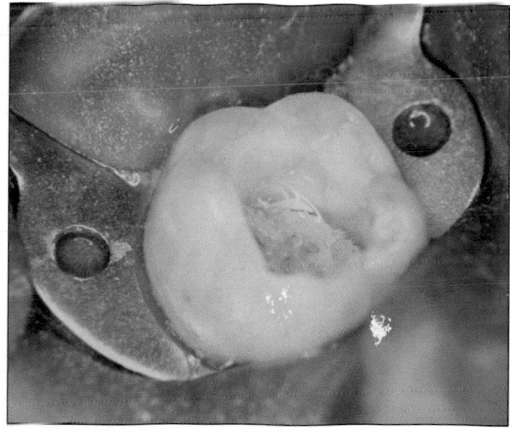

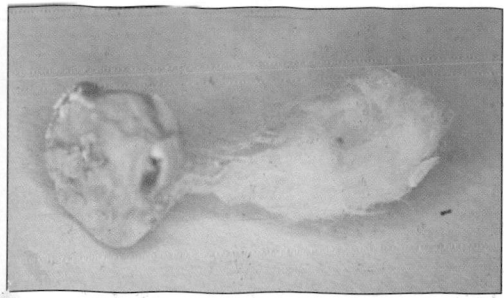

Fig. 16 A layer of gutta-percha temporary filling material has been placed to protect the root canals before the restorative material is applied. The inset shows how this may be removed and prevents fragments of the temporary filling entering the root canal.

1. Mullaney T P. Instrumentation of finely curved canals. *Dent Clin North Am* 1979; **23**: 575–592.
2. Goerig A C, Michelich R J, Schult H H. Instrumentation of root canals in molars using the stepdown technique. *J Endod* 1982; **8**: 550–554.
3. Fava L R. The double flared technique: an alternative for biomechanical preparation. *J Endod* 1983; **9**: 76–80.
4. Morgan L F, Montgomery S. An evaluation of the crown-down pressureless technique. *J Endod* 1984; **10**: 491–498.
5. Abou-Rass M, Frank A, Glick D. The anticurvature filing method to prepare the curved root canal. *J Am Dent Assoc* 1980; **101**: 792–794.
6. Roane J B, Sabala C L, Duncanson M G. The 'balanced force' concept for instrumentation of curved canals. *J Endod* 1985; **11**: 203–211.
7. Ahmad M, Pitt Ford T, Crum L. Ultrasonic debridement of root canals: an insight into the mechanisms involved. *J Endod* 1987; **13**: 93–101.
8. Griffiths B, Stock C. The efficiency of irrigants in removing root canal debris when used with an ultrasonic preparation technique. *Int Endod J* 1986; **19**: 277–284.
9. Sabala C L, Powell S E. Sodium hypochlorite injection into periapical tissues. *J Endod* 1989; **15**: 490–492
10. Berutti E, Marini R, A scanning electron microscope evaluation of the debridement capability of sodium hypochlorite at different temperatures. *J Endod* 1996; **22**: 467–470.
11. Pagavino G, Pace R, Baccetti T. A SEM study of in vivo accuracy of the Root ZX electronic apex locator. *J Endod* 1998; **24**: 438–441.
12. McDonald N J. The electronic determination of working length. *Dent Clin North Am* 1992; **36**: 293–307.
13. Lumley P J. Management of silver points and fractured instruments. *CPD Dentistry* 2000; **1**: 87–92.
14. Buchanan L S. The art of endodontics: Files of greater taper. *Dentistry Today* 1996; **42**: 44–49.
15. Kavanagh D, Lumley P J. An in vitro evaluation of canal preparation using Profile .04 and .06 taper instruments. *Endod Dent Traumatol* 1998; **14**: 16–20.
16. Hulsmann M, Schade M, Schafers F. A comparative study of root canal preparation with HERO 642 and Quantec SC rotary Ni-Ti instruments. *Int Endod J* 2001; **34**: 538–546.
17. Barbakow F, Lutz F. The Lightspeed preparation technique evaluated by Swiss clinicians after attending continuing education courses. *Int Endod J* 1997; **30**: 46–50.
18. Bryant S T, Thompson S A, Al-Omari M A, Dummer P M H. Shaping ability of Profile rotary nickel-titanium instruments with ISO sized tips in simulated root canals. *Int Endod J* 1998; **31**: (part 1) 275–281, (part 2) 282–289.
19. Buchanan L S. The standardised taper root canal preparation. Parts 1–6. *Int Endod J*. Part 1 2000; **33**: 516–529; Part 2 2001; **34**: 63–71; Part 3 2001; **34**: 149–156; Part 4 2001; **34**: 157–164; Part 5 2001; **34**: 244–249; Part 6 2001; **34**: 250–259;
20. Ruddle C J. in Cohen S and Burns R C, *Pathways of the Pulp* Eighth Edition, Page 276–277. St Louis: Mosby, 2002.
21. Sjögren U, Figdor D, Persson S, Sundqvist G. Influence of infection at the time of root filling on the outcome or endodontic treatment of teeth with apical periodontitis. *Int Endod J* 1997; **30**: 297–306.
22. Guttman J L. Presentation to The British Endodontic Society Spring Scientific Meeting, October 2000, Chester, UK.
23. Anderson R W, Powell B J, Pashley D H. Microleakage of three temporary endodontic restorations. *J Endod* 1988; **14**: 497–501.

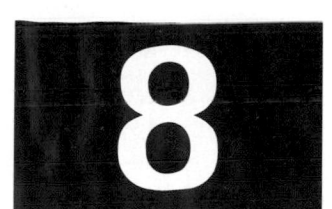
IN BRIEF

- No matter how well the obturation of the root canals is performed, success will be dependant upon the initial cleaning and debridement of the entire root canal system.
- Cold lateral compaction of a master gutta percha point and accessory points remains the norm against which other obturation methods are assessed.
- The gold standard of obturation is the warm vertical compaction of gutta percha with a heated plugger.
- Research suggests that the coronal seal, achieved with a layer of glass ionomer cement on the floor of the pulp chamber, may be more important than the apical seal.

Filling the root canal system

The purpose of the obturation phase of a root filling is two-fold; to prevent microorganisms from re-entering the root canal system, and to isolate any microorganisms that may remain within the tooth from nutrients in tissue fluids. The seal at the apical end of the root canal is achieved by a well-fitting gutta-percha master point, and accessory points, although heated techniques may result in a better seal. The seal at the coronal end is achieved by the application of a layer of resin-modified glass ionomer cement as accessory canals may lead from the floor of the pulp chamber to the furcation area. It must always be remembered that success will only be achieved if the root canal system has been as thoroughly debrided as possible of infected material.

In modern endodontic treatment the emphasis is placed far more on cleaning and preparing the root canal system than on filling it. This does not mean that root canal obturation is less important, but that the success of endodontic treatment depends on meticulous root canal preparation.

The purpose of a root canal filling, as illustrated in Figure 1, is to seal the root canal system to prevent:

- Microorganisms from entering and reinfecting the root canal system;
- Tissue fluids from percolating back into the root canal system and providing a culture medium for any residual bacteria.[1]

In the past, attention has been focussed on the importance of obtaining an hermetic apical seal. However, research has indicated that as well as sealing the root canal system apically, it is equally important to ensure that the coronal access to the canal itself has a fluid-tight seal, to prevent infection from the oral cavity.[2] Although numerous materials have been used to fill root canals, the most universally accepted is gutta-percha.

PROPERTIES OF ROOT CANAL FILLING MATERIALS[1]

Ideally, a root canal filling should be:

- Biocompatible.
- Dimensionally stable.
- Capable of sealing the canal laterally and apically, conforming with the various shapes and contours of the individual canal.
- Unaffected by tissue fluids and insoluble.

- Bacteriostatic.
- Radiopaque.
- Easily removed from the canal if necessary.

To these properties may also be added, incapable of staining tooth or gingival tissues and easily manipulated with ample working time.

Gutta-percha has a number of these desirable properties. It is semisolid and can be compressed and packed to fill the irregular shapes of a root canal using lateral or vertical compaction techniques. It is non-irritant and dimensionally stable. It will become plastic when heated or when used with solvents (xylol, chloroform, eucalyptus oil).

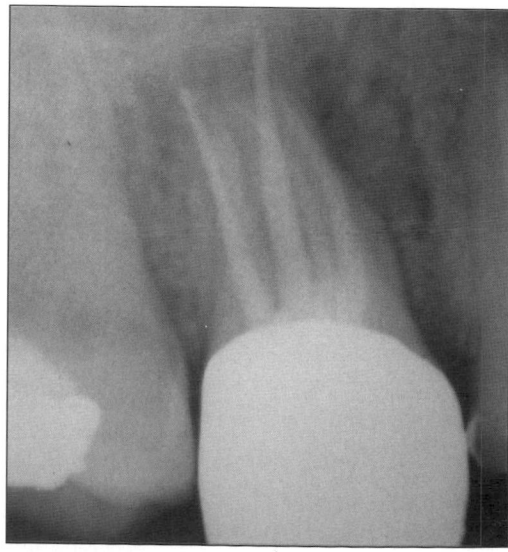

Fig. 1 A radiograph of a well–obturated upper molar.

Fig. 2 These teeth with resorptive defects may be impossible to obturate with conventional methods.

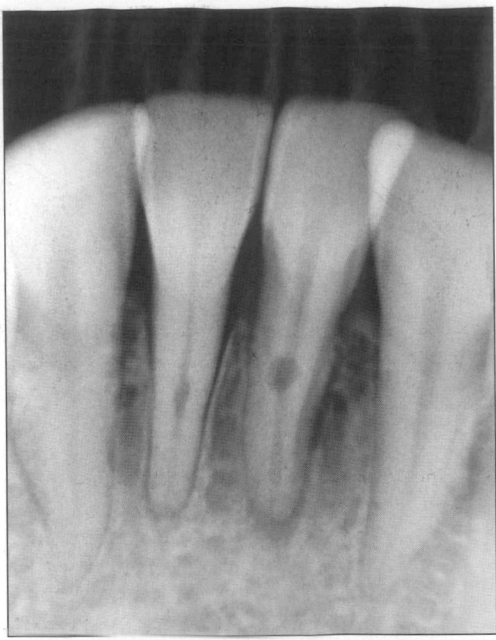

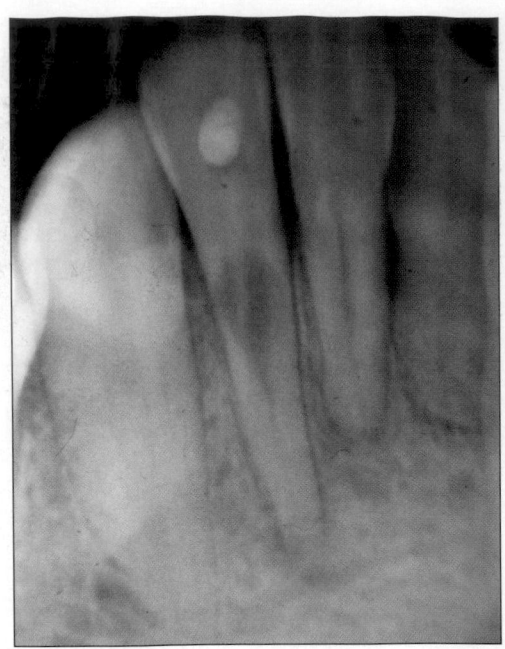

It is radiopaque and inert, and can be removed from the canal when required for post preparation.

Its disadvantages are few. It is distorted by pressure and, consequently, can be forced through the apical foramen if too much pressure is used, and it is not rigid and so can be difficult to use in smaller sizes. Also, a sealer is necessary to fill in the spaces around the filling material. Root canal scalers wre considered in Part 5.

Gutta-percha points are manufactured in various forms. Standardized points match the ISO sizes, and have a 2% taper. Accessory points have fine tips and variable taper to facilitate and improve lateral compaction. Greater taper points are available in 4% and 6% taper to match modern preparation techniques. Feather-tipped points permit individual and specific cone fitting to the prepared root canal.

REMOVAL OF SMEAR LAYER

A smear layer is created by the action of metallic instruments on dentine, especially rotary instruments. It is composed of dentine filings, pulpal tissue remnants and may also contain microbial elements. It may occlude dentine tubules thus harbouring bacteria, and may contain a bacterial plaque on the canal walls. It has been shown that gutta-percha penetrates the dentine tubules when the smear layer has been removed.[3]

It is therefore suggested that the root canal should be irrigated with an EDTA solution to remove the smear layer, followed by a final irrigation with sodium hypochlorite, prior to drying and obturating the canal.

FILLING TECHNIQUES

The studious reader will have noted the use of the word 'compaction' rather than 'condensation'. In 1998, the American Endodontic Association recognized that this was a more appropriate term for the techniques used in obturation, and the term has been adopted in this text.[4]

Several techniques have been developed for placing gutta-percha into the root canal system. Nevertheless, the cold lateral compaction of gutta-percha is still the most widely taught, and the technique against which most others are compared. However, as there is a demand for saving teeth with complex pathology and root canal morphology (Fig. 2), it is sometimes easier to combine the merits of various techniques in a hybrid form to simplify the filling procedure. Studies have shown that these are satisfactory, although not always as easy as lateral compaction to carry out.[5,6]

Before a root-filling is inserted, it is essential that the canals are dry. Any serous exudate from the periapical tissues indicates the presence of inflammation. Calcium hydroxide may be used as a root canal dressing until the next visit (calcium hydroxide BP mixed with purified water or local anaesthetic solution to a thick paste – see Part 9).

LATERAL COMPACTION OF GUTTA–PERCHA

The objective is to fill the canal with gutta-percha points (cones) by compacting them laterally against the sides of the canal walls. The technique requires selection of a master point, usually one size larger than the master apical file, which should seat about 0.5 mm short of the working length (Fig. 3a). If the point is loose at working length, then either 1 mm should be cut from the tip and the point refitted to the canal, or a larger size point selected. It should be noted that gutta-percha points can not be as accurately machined as metallic instruments. There may be variance in the size stated, and if a matched point does not fit a prepared canal it may be worth either trying another point from the packet, or fitting the point in a measuring/sizing gauge, as illustrated in Figure 4.

Once the master point is fitted to length and demonstrates a slight resistance to withdrawal (tug-back), accessory points are then inserted

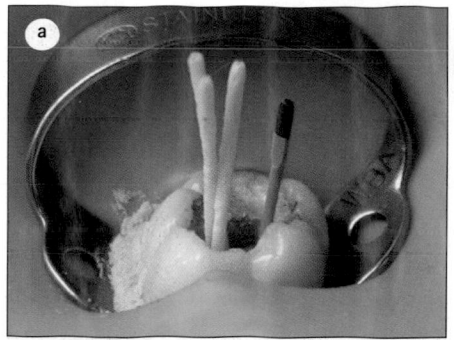
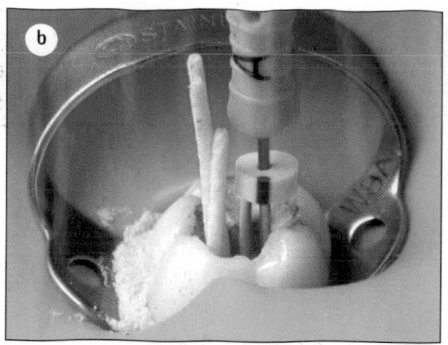
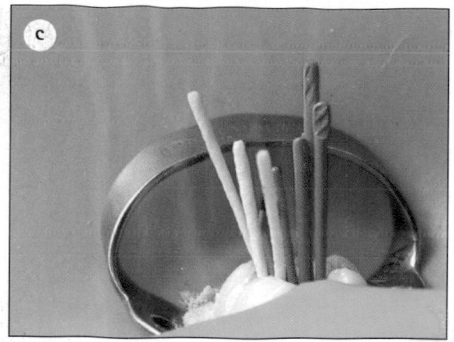

Fig. 3 a) In cold lateral compaction, the master point should exhibit 'tug-back' slightly short of the working lengths. (Paper points have been placed to protect the other canals.) b) A finger spreader inserted alongside the master point, is left in place for 30 seconds. c) The spiral of successive accessory points in an effective obturation.

alongside the master point and compacted laterally with a spreader until the canal is sealed (Fig. 3b). The most simple system of accessory points designates these from A, the finest, through B and C to D, the largest, shown in Figure 5. As each point is used the prepared, flared, canal is becoming progressively wider, and the accessory points may therefore be used sequentially from small to large. The resultant filling appears above the access cavity as a spiral, with each point extruded slightly further out of the canal (Fig. 3c).

There are two main types of spreading instruments for compacting gutta-percha: long-handled spreaders and finger spreaders. The main advantage of a finger spreader is that it is not possible to exert the high lateral pressure that might occur with long-handled spreaders. The chance of a root fracture is reduced and it is therefore a suitable instrument for beginners.

PROCEDURE

1. The canal should be irrigated, cleaned and dried.
2. A master point is selected and fitted to the canal as described above. It should be marked at working length, or grasped securely in endodontic locking tweezers.

3. The master point is coated with sealer and used to paste the canal walls with the sealer, using an in-out movement, before seating the point home into the canal at full working length.
4. A fine finger spreader is selected and the rubber stop set to working length. Place the spreader alongside the master point and compact using firm apical finger pressure only. Leave the spreader in situ for 30 seconds. This is important as continuous pressure from the spreader is required to deform the gutta-percha point against the canal walls and to overcome its elasticity.
5. Select an accessory point with locking tweezers and dip its tip into sealer. Do not leave the points in sealer while working (Fig. 6) as a reaction may occur between the zinc oxide in the points (up to 80%) and the eugenol in the sealer, softening the points and making insertion difficult.
6. This stage is best carried out using two hands. Assuming the operator is right handed, the tweezers holding the accessory point are aligned above the tooth in the right hand, while the left hand rotates the spreader a few times through an arc of 30–40° and withdraws it.

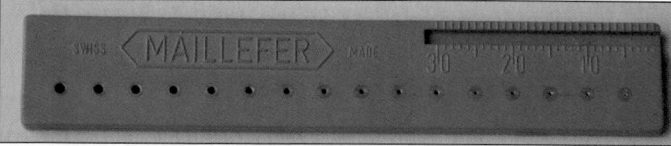

Fig. 4 An endodontic gauge for accurately sizing gutta–percha points.

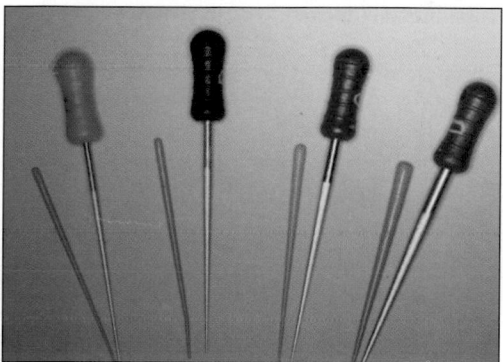

Fig. 5 Finger spreaders sized A to D with matching accessory points.

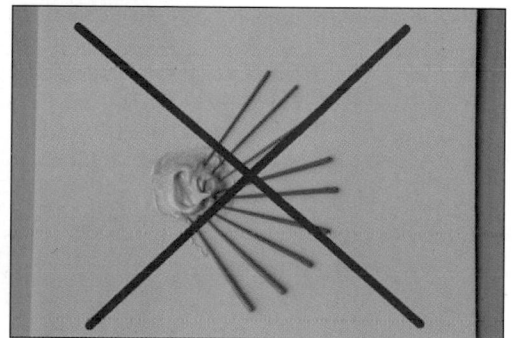

Fig. 6 Gutta–percha points should NOT be presented to the operator by the surgery assistant with the tips dipped in sealer.

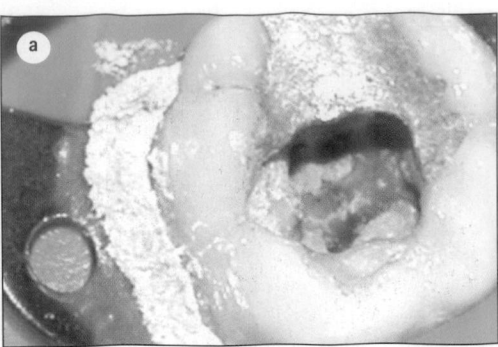
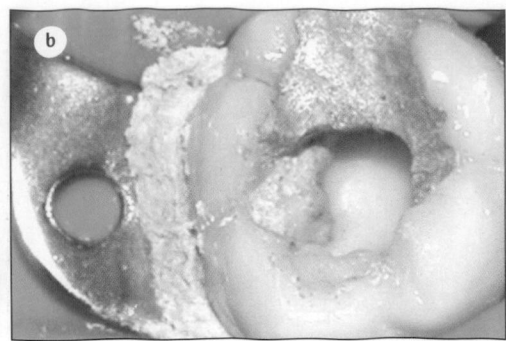

Fig. 7 The excess gutta-percha has been removed with a hot instrument, and the coronal filling has been compacted into the root canal orifice a), prior to the placement of a glass ionomer coronal seal b).

7. Immediately place the accessory point alongside the master point. Any delay will allow the master point to relax and space will be lost. Reinsert the spreader and laterally compact both points.

8. Repeat the sequence using gradually larger spreaders and gutta-percha points until the canal is filled.

9. Remove excess gutta-percha from the canal orifice with a heated plugger, and firmly compact the remaining gutta-percha to seal the coronal access to the canal (Fig. 7).

10. If post-space preparation is required it may be carried out at this stage.

11. If not, a layer of resin-modified glass-ionomer cement should be applied over the gutta-percha and the floor of the access cavity, completing the coronal seal.

12. A periapical radiograph should be taken on completion, using a long-cone parallel technique. This is primarily for subsequent monitoring of healing by sequential radiographs, taken if possible in the same film-holder system to ensure reproducible and comparable exposures.

LATERAL COMPACTION OF WARM GUTTA–PERCHA

A simple modification to the cold lateral compaction technique is to apply heat to the gutta-percha. The softened material is easier to compact and will result in a denser root filling. However, finger spreaders will not retain heat sufficiently for this procedure, and specially designed heat carriers should be used. The instruments illustrated in Figure 8 have a sharp tip for lateral compaction, and a blunt plugger tip for limited vertical compaction of the softened gutta-percha. Electrically heated spreaders are also available. It is important that the instruments are only gently warmed. If the spreader is too hot it will melt the gutta-percha, which will adhere to the instrument and be withdrawn from the canal.

SINGLE GUTTA–PERCHA POINT AND SEALER

With the tendency to preparation techniques of greater taper, gutta-percha points of matching taper may be used. These fit the prepared canal so well that some operators are using a single gutta-percha point and sealer. The only advantage of this technique is its simplicity. The disadvantage is that the majority of sealers are soluble. As the canal will not be fully filled in three dimensions, tissue fluids may leach out the sealer over time. This technique cannot therefore be recommended.

However, in difficult anatomical cases it may be necessary to create a custom-fitted cone. A slightly large cone is selected and the apical part softened, either by solvents such as chloroform, rectified turpentine or oil of eucalyptus, or by immersion in hot water. The softened cone is fitted to working length with gentle pressure. The cone is carefully marked for orientation, and the process repeated until a satisfactory fit is obtained. The cone should then be cleaned of all solvents, and the canal obturated using sealer in the usual way.

As with all single-cone techniques, if the excess sealer resorbs in the apical tissue fluids, microleakage may allow the ingress of tissue fluids, and failure of the stated criteria of obturation. Really, an attempt should always be made to improve the fit of a single cone with warm or cold lateral compaction of accessory points.

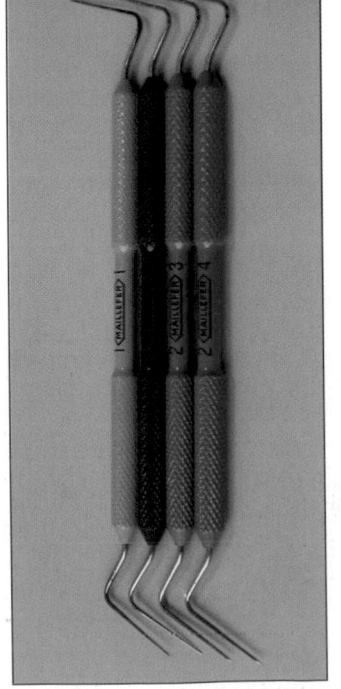

Fig. 8 Machtou heat carriers/pluggers for warm compaction.

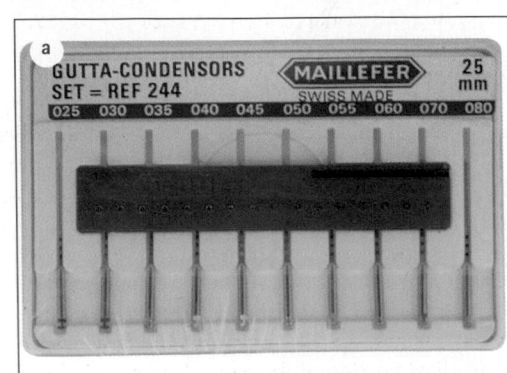

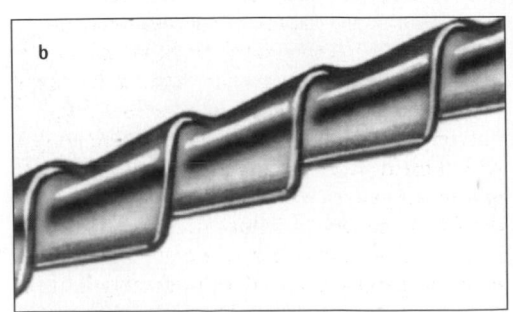

Fig. 9 a) Maillefer Gutta Condensors, with b) showing the apically directed thread structure.

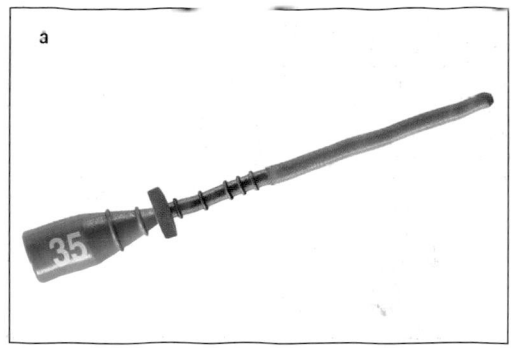

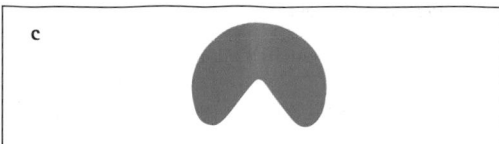

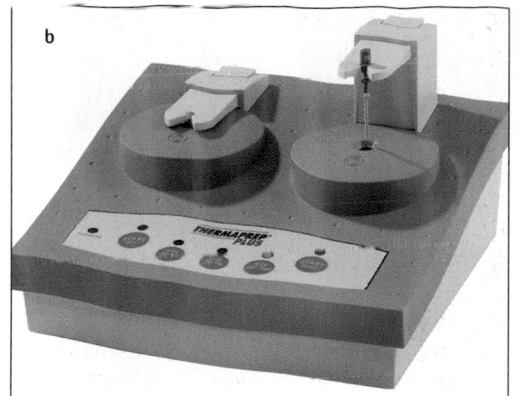

Fig. 10 An example of a Thermafil device a), a heated gutta-percha carrier, with an oven necessary for accurate softening b). The U-shaped cross-section of the plastic carrier is shown in c).

THERMATIC COMPACTION OF GUTTA-PERCHA

In 1979, McSpadden devised a handpiece-driven compactor, which is effectively an inverted Hedstroem file.[7] Although no longer made, other similar devices, such as the gutta condensor (Fig. 9), are available. The frictional heat from the compactor plasticizes the gutta-percha and the blades drive the softened material into the root canal under pressure. The main problem found was lack of control over the apical portion of the gutta-percha, which may be extruded through the apex in its softened state. To overcome this problem, the technique was modified by Tagger, who recommended laterally condensing a master point and two or three accessory points, and then using the condensor to plasticize the gutta-percha in the coronal part of the canal.[8] The laterally compacted material in the apical half effectively prevents any apical extrusion.

The technique is particularly useful for the rapid and effective obturation of the coronal part of a root canal after placement of an accurate apical seal.

HEATED GUTTA-PERCHA CARRIERS

Several manufacturers now supply these devices, illustrated in Figure 10. Alpha-phase gutta-percha is attached to a rigid carrier, in a variation of the technique originally described by Johnson in 1978.[9] Most carriers are now plastic. The excess material is removed, and the carrier remains in the canal as a central core. The softened gutta-percha flows well in to canal aberrations, fins, etc., giving very good three-dimensional obturation.[10] Success depends, as with all techniques, upon thorough canal cleaning and shaping. The carriers have a 4% taper, and an underprepared canal will be difficult if not impossible to obturate to working length with these devices. A range of sizes is presented, and most systems employ a method of ensuring the fit of the device before obturation is commenced. This may either be a blank carrier with no gutta-percha attached, or preferably a file of the same dimensions as the carrier. The apical preparation may then be refined to ensure an accurate fit of the device.

The canal should be cleaned and dried, and a very fine coating of sealer applied to the canal orifice only. Excess sealer may be extruded under hydraulic pressure through the apical foramen, with resultant pain and inflammation. In the meantime the rubber stop on the selected device is set to working length, and the device placed in a special oven to soften the gutta-percha. When ready, the device should be swiftly and smoothly inserted to working length, and held in place for a few seconds. Using a high-speed bur the excess carrier may be sectioned and removed from the canal orifice, and a plugger used to compact the gutta-percha in this area. A layer of resin-modified glass ionomer completes the obturation.

Some carriers are manufactured with a U-shaped cross-section to facilitate removal with a drill should retreatment be necessary. However, although it may be possible to drill out the carrier, this technique may not be appropriate if a post and core may be indicated in the future.

VERTICAL COMPACTION OF WARM GUTTA-PERCHA

Heated gutta-percha has been shown to flow extremely well into all canal irregularities. It is particularly useful in situations such as internal resorption, C-shaped canals, and those with fins or webs. As referred to earlier, when the smear layer is removed the gutta-percha has been shown to penetrate dentine tubules.[3] This technique is now considered the gold standard for endodontic obturation. The principle of vertical compaction of increments of warm gutta-percha was first described by Schilder in 1967.[11] Although delivering excellent results, the method was difficult to master and time-consuming.

The state of the art at present is the method first described by Buchanan employing the System-B heat source (Fig. 11), which delivers a precise heat to the tip of the plugger.[12] A non-standardized (4%, 6% or feathered tip) gutta-percha cone is carefully fitted to the canal. Using a selected plugger, a continuous wave of heat is applied to soften and downpack a cone, resulting in very well-compacted obturation of the apical portion of the canal. The remainder of

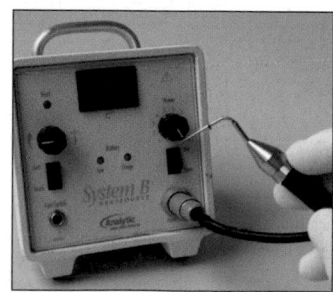

Fig. 11 The System-B heat source. When the ring on the handpiece is pressed as shown the tip of the plugger is immediately heated to the temperature selected.

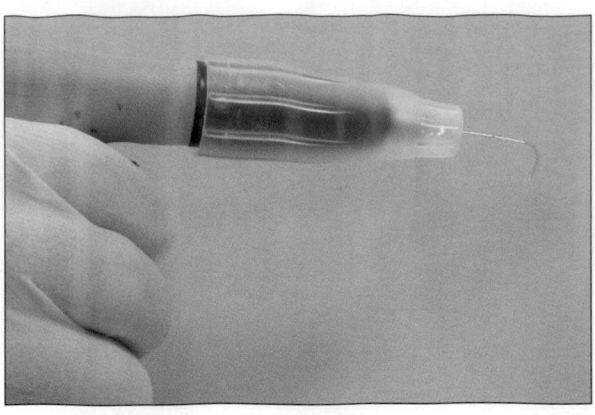

Fig. 12 Heated alpha-phase gutta-percha being extruded from the silver needle of the Obtura II machine.

the canal may be obturated by further increments, or by another method. Briefly, the technique is as follows.

1. Fit a gutta-percha cone and mark it at working length.
2. Select one of the System-B pluggers that binds in the canal 5–7 mm short of the working length. Set a rubber stop at this level, and select a conventional plugger to fit at this length as well.
3. Dry the canal with paper points.
4. Apply a thin layer of sealer to the apical third of the selected cone, and insert it to working length.
5. Set the temperature of the System-B at 200°C, with full power. Heat is applied to the plugger via the finger-tip microswitch, and the part of the cone extruding from the canal orifice is seared off.
6. The tip of the plugger is placed in the centre of the gutta-percha cone, heat applied, and the plugger is carefully pushed down the canal in one slow, even movement to the depth marked. This should take about 3 seconds. The heat is turned off, and the plugger held in place for a further 10 seconds.
7. With a brief burst of heat to separate the plugger from the gutta-percha, the plugger is removed from the canal. It is usually found to bring with it the coronal portion of the gutta-percha as well.
8. The apical part may now be further compacted with conventional hand pluggers.
9. The coronal part of the canal may now be obturated with either injectable gutta-percha, described later, or further use of the System-B as follows.
10. A small length of gutta-percha, about 7 mm, is cut from a further accessory point, coated with sealer and inserted into the canal.
11. With the heat source turned down to 100°C, otherwise this gutta-percha will not stay in the canal, a short burst of heat is applied, the gutta-percha compacted, and the plugger removed as before. Hand pluggers may be used to further compact this and any subsequent increments required.
12. A layer of resin-modified glass-ionomer cement is applied over the obturation, and a post-operative radiograph is exposed as normal.

INJECTABLE GUTTA–PERCHA

Devices for injecting softened gutta-percha have been available for some time, but in the past have suffered from techniques which led to difficulty in accurate apical placement. The latest of these, the Obtura-II, has recently gained acceptance by endodontists. The machine resembles a glue-gun. Pellets of alpha-phase gutta-percha are softened at about 200°C in the handpiece, and extruded through a heated silver needle (Fig. 11). A wide, well-prepared canal is a prerequisite. Although the manufacturers describe a procedure for total obturation of a root canal, apical control can be difficult. The machine has become accepted for two specific procedures.

CORONAL BACK–FILLING

The previously described System-B achieves an excellent and controlled obturation of the apical 5–7 mm of the root canal. At this point the canal is quite wide, and can accept the tip of the Obtura's needle. A film of sealer is applied to the canal wall. The machine is heated to 200°C. A small amount of the warm gutta-percha should be extruded to warm the needle and discarded. The needle is then quickly introduced to the canal. If this part of the protocol is not followed, a void may result between the two parts of the filling. The trigger is activated and thermoplasticized gutta-percha extruded into the canal, gently pushing the needle out. Once the canal is filled conventional pluggers may be used to compact the gutta-percha, which is finally sealed with glass ionomer as usual.

OPEN APICES

The open apex, particularly in paediatric endodontics, can present a problem if it is too wide to permit the creation of a custom-fitted cone. A method of using the Obtura-II has been described whereby an increment of gutta-percha is applied to the canal close to the apex, and gently compacted with pluggers. A rapid-developing radiograph is exposed to verify the position of the apical seal, and further compaction carried out if required. Once the apical seal is intact the remainder of the canal may be filled with the Obtura-II in the normal way.

1. European Society of Endodontology. Consensus report for the European Society of Endodontology on quality guidelines for endodontic treatment. *Int Endod J* 1994; **27**: 115–124.
2. Saunders W P, Saunders E M. Coronal leakage as a cause of failure in root canal therapy: a review. *Endod Dent Traumatol* 1994; **10**: 105–108.
3. Gutmann J L. Adaptation of injected thermoplasticised gutta percha in the absence of the dentinal smear layer. *Int Endod J* 1993; **26**: 87–92.
4. American Association of Endodontists. *Glossary, contemporary terminology for endodontics*, edition 6. Chicago: American Association of Endodontists, 1998.
5. Gee J Y. A comparison of five methods of root canal obturation by dye penetration. *Aust Dent J* 1987; **32**: 279–284.
6. Haas S B, Campbell A D, Hicks M L, Pelleu G B. A comparison of four root canal filling techniques. *J Endod* 1989; **15**: 596–601.
7. McSpadden J T. Presentation to the meeting of the American Association of Endodontists, Atlanta, Georgia, USA 1979.

8. Jagger M, Tanse A, Katz A, Korzen B H. Evaluation of the apical seal produced by a hybrid root canal filling method, combining lateral condensation and thermal compaction. *J Endod* 1984; 10: 299–303.

9. Johnson W B. A new gutta-percha technique. *J Endod* 1978; 4: 184–188.

10. Gutman J L, Saunders W P, Saunders E M, Nguyen L. An assessment of the plastic thermal obturation technique. II Material adaptation and sealability. *Int Endod J* 1993; 26: 179–183.

11. Schilder H. Filling root canals in three dimensions. *Dent Clin North Am* 1967; 11: 723–744.

12. Buchanan L S. The continuous wave of obturation technique: 'centred' condensation of warm gutta percha in 12 seconds. *Dent Today* 1996; 15: 60–87.

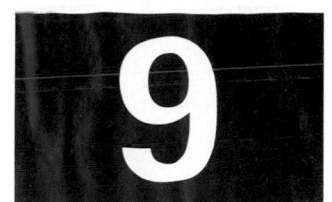

IN BRIEF
- Calcium hydroxide is used in both the preservation of the vital pulp and the disinfection of the prepared root canal system
- To achieve success in direct pulp capping a strict aseptic regime must be followed.
- Various forms of root resorption, their aetiology and treatment, are considered
- The Simon, Glick and Frank classification of endodontic/periodontic lesions is presented and discussed.

Calcium hydroxide, root resorption, endo-perio lesions

For more than 70 years calcium hydroxide has played a major role in endodontic therapy, although many of its functions are now being taken over by the recently introduced material MTA. Calcium hydroxide may be used to preserve the vital pulp if infection and bleeding are controlled; to repair root fractures, perforations, open apices and root resorptions. Endo-perio lesions are complex and the correct diagnosis is essential if treatment is to be successful. However, root canal treatment will always be the first phase in treating such lesions.

CALCIUM HYDROXIDE

Calcium hydroxide was originally introduced to the field of endodontics by Herman[1] in 1930 as a pulp-capping agent, but its uses today are widespread in endodontic therapy. It is the most commonly used dressing for treatment of the vital pulp. It also plays a major role as an inter-visit dressing in the disinfection of the root canal system.

Mode of action

A calcified barrier may be induced when calcium hydroxide is used as a pulp-capping agent or placed in the root canal in contact with healthy pulpal or periodontal tissue. Because of the high pH of the material, up to 12.5, a superficial layer of necrosis occurs in the pulp to a depth of up to 2 mm. Beyond this layer only a mild inflammatory response is seen, and providing the operating field was kept free of bacteria when the material was placed, a hard tissue barrier may be formed. However, the calcium ions that form the barrier are derived entirely from the bloodstream and not from the calcium hydroxide.[2] The hydroxyl group is considered to be the most important component of calcium hydroxide as it provides an alkaline environment which encourages repair and active calcification. The alkaline pH induced not only neutralizes lactic acid from the osteoclasts, thus preventing a dissolution of the mineral components of dentine, but could also activate alkaline phosphatases which play an important role in hard tissue formation. The calcified material which is produced appears to be the product of both odontoblasts and connective tissue cells and may be termed osteodentine. The barrier, which is composed of osteodentine, is not always complete and is porous.

In external resorption, the cementum layer is lost from a portion of the root surface, which allows communication through the dentinal tubules between the root canal and the periodontal tissues. It has been shown that the disassociation coefficient of calcium hydroxide of 0.17 permits a slow, controlled release of both calcium and hydroxyl ions which can diffuse through dentinal tubules. Tronstad et al. demonstrated that untreated teeth with pulpal necrosis had a pH of 6.0 to 7.4 in the pulp dentine and periodontal ligament, whereas, after calcium hydroxide had been placed in the canals, the teeth showed a pH range in the peripheral dentine of 7.4 to 9.6.[3]

Tronstad et al. suggest that calcium hydroxide may have other actions; these include, for example, arresting inflammatory root resorption and stimulation of healing.[3] It also has a bactericidal effect and will denature proteins found in the root canal, thereby making them less toxic. Finally, calcium ions are an integral part of the immunological reaction and may activate the calcium-dependent adenosine triphosphatase reaction associated with hard tissue formation.

Presentation

Calcium hydroxide can be applied as a hard setting cement, as a paste or as a powder/liquid mixture, depending on the treatment. Various proprietary brands are available, (Fig. 1), although ordinary calcium hydroxide powder BP

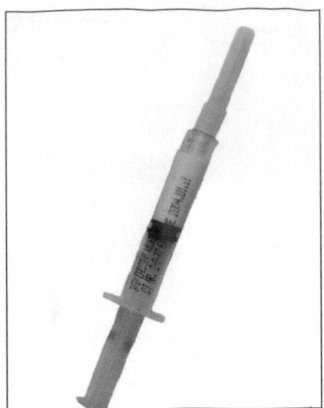

Fig. 1 One of various proprietary brands of calcium hydroxide available.

may be purchased from a chemist and mixed with purified water. Because of the antibacterial effect of calcium hydroxide, it is not necessary to add a germicide. The advantages of using calcium hydroxide in this form are that variable consistencies may be mixed and a pH of about 12 is achieved, which is higher than that of proprietary brands.

Root canal sealers containing calcium hydroxide are available, and are discussed in Part 5.

Clinical uses and techniques

The clinical situations where calcium hydroxide may be used in endodontics are discussed below and the techniques described. The method of application of calcium hydroxide to tissue is important if the maximum benefit is to be gained. When performing pulp capping, pulpotomy or treatment to an open apex in a pulpless tooth, the exposed tissue should be cleaned thoroughly, any haemorrhage arrested by irrigation with sterile saline and the use of sterile cotton wool pledgets. The calcium hydroxide should be placed gently directly on to the tissue, with no debris or blood intervening.[4] A calcium hydroxide cement may be applied to protect the pulp in a deep cavity as discussed later.

Routine canal medication

The indications for intervisit dressing of the root canal with calcium hydroxide have been considered in Part 7. There are two methods of inserting calcium hydroxide paste into the root canal, the object being to fill the root canal completely with calcium hydroxide so that it is in contact with healthy tissue. Care should be taken to prevent the extrusion of paste into the periapical tissues, although if this does occur healing will not be seriously affected.

Proprietary brands

The root canal system is first prepared and then dried. A spiral root canal filler is selected and passively tried in the canal. It must be a loose fit in the canal over its entire length, or fracture may occur, as seen in Figure 2. The working length of the canal should be marked on the shank with either marking paste or a rubber stop. The author prefers the blade type of filler

as these are less prone to fracture. The paste of choice is spread evenly on the shank. The spiral filler is inserted into the canal and 'wiped' around the walls to reduce air bubble formation. Using a standard handpiece with low rpm, the root canal is filled with paste. Several applications may be required. A large paper point may be used to condense the material into the canal, and this will also absorb excess moisture. A pledget of cotton wool is pressed into the pulp chamber so that the paste is condensed further and the access cavity sealed.

Powder—liquid

The powder and liquid are mixed on a glass slab with a spatula to form a thick paste. Although sterile water may be used, local anaesthetic solution is more readily available in the surgery. The material may be applied using a spiral root canal filler as described earlier, however some practitioners prefer to use the small plastic tube with a long fine point illustrated in Part 7, Figure 14. The mixed material is loaded into the tube and extruded directly deep in the canal. A large paper point may again be used to condense the material further, and absorb excess water making the procedure easier and the filling more dense (Fig. 3). A firmer paste may be made by adding powder to a proprietary brand of calcium hydroxide paste.

Of utmost importance in endodontics is the temporary coronal seal which prevents leakage and (re)contamination of the canal system. Intermediate restorative material (IRM), or glass-ionomer cement are useful for periods of over 7–10 days; for shorter periods, zinc oxide, Cavit or other proprietary material may be used, as described in Part 5.

Radiographic appearance

A root canal filled with calcium hydroxide should appear on a radiograph as if it were completely sclerosed, as in Figure 4. The material is prone to dissolution, which would appear on a radiograph as voids in the canal. In the past, the addition of more radiopaque agents such as barium sulphate has been recommended. As these materials may be resorbed more slowly than the calcium hydroxide a false picture may be given, and this practice has largely been discontinued.

Indirect pulp capping

The treatment of the deep carious lesion which has not yet involved the pulp has for some time been the subject of intense debate. Some researchers recommend the use of a calcium hydroxide lining to stimulate odontoblasts and increase dentine formation.[4,5] Other workers have claimed that this does not occur.[6,7] Some workers still recommend that infected carious dentine is removed but a layer of softened sterile dentine may be left over the intact vital pulp.[8] Most endodontic texts, (for example, see References 9 and 10) recommend that all softened dentine should be removed and the pulp dealt with accordingly.

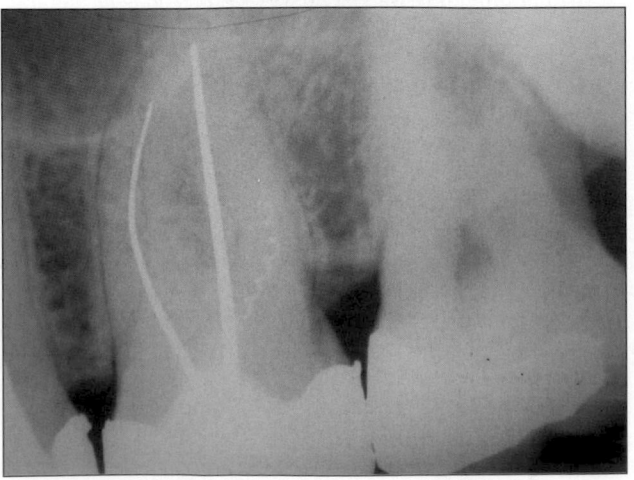

Fig. 2 Spiral root fillers are prone to fracture if their passive fit in the root canal has not been verified before use.

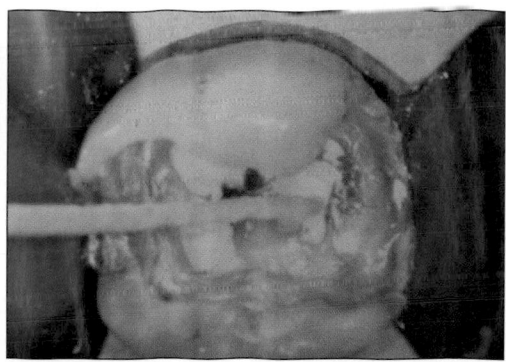

Fig. 3 A paper point may be used to condense the calcium hydroxide in the canal and remove excess moisture.

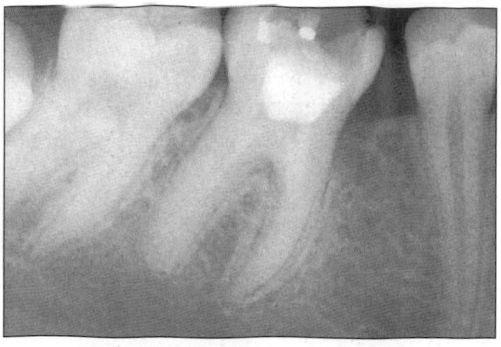

Fig. 4 A radiograph showing root canal system filled with calcium hydroxide, which has the same radio-density as the dentine. Any part of the canal not filled with the paste appears as a void.

There is still controversy, however, over the correct treatment of a deep, caries free, cavity, lying close to the pulp. As alluded to in Part 1, the essential treatment is to ensure that there can be no bacterial contamination of the pulp via the exposed dentine tubules.[11] This may be achieved by either a lining of glass-ionomer cement, or the use of an acid-etched dentine bonding system. Some workers have recommended washing the cavity with sodium hypochlorite to further disinfect the dentine surface, and this seems an eminently sensible suggestion. Until further research provides conclusive evidence for or against, however, the use of an indirect pulp cap of calcium hydroxide is recommended in these situations. The calcium hydroxide cement provides a bactericidal effect on any remaining bacteria and may encourage the formation of secondary dentine and of a dentine bridge. It is certainly no longer considered necessary to reopen the cavity at a later date to confirm healing.

Direct pulp capping

The aim of direct pulp capping is to protect the vital pulp which has been exposed during cavity preparation, either through caries or trauma. The most important consideration in obtaining success is that the pulp tissue remains uncontaminated. In deep cavities, when an exposure may be anticipated, all caries should be removed before approaching the pulpal aspect of the cavity floor. If an exposure of the pulp occurs in a carious field the chances of successful pulp capping are severely compromised. A rubber dam should be applied as soon as pulp capping is proposed. The pulp should be symptom-free and uninfected, and the exposure should be small. Before commencing large restorations in suspicious teeth it may be prudent to test the vitality of the tooth with an electronic pulp tester, and also to expose a radiograph to ensure that there is no evidence of pulpal or periapical pathology. The radiograph may in fact be more valuable, as misleading results may occur when using an electric pulp tester on compromised multirooted teeth.

If the above criteria have been met and pulp capping is indicated, the cavity should be cleaned thoroughly, ideally with sodium hypochlorite solution, and pulpal haemorrhage arrested with sterile cotton pledgets. Persistent bleeding indicates an inflamed pulp, which may not respond to treatment. After placing the calcium hydroxide, the area must be sealed against bacterial ingress, preferably with a glass-ionomer lining.

Partial pulpotomy

Although the technique of pulpotomy is indicated for immature teeth with open apices, as described in Part 10, it cannot be recommended routinely in mature teeth. However, the technique of partial pulpotomy (a procedure between pulp capping and pulpotomy) was introduced by Cvek and has been shown to be very successful in the treatment of traumatically exposed pulps.[12,13] The exposed pulp and surrounding dentine is removed under rubber dam isolation with a high-speed diamond drill and copious irrigation using sterile saline, to a depth of about 2 mm. Haemostasis is achieved and the wound dressed with a non-setting calcium hydroxide paste, either powder and sterile saline or a proprietary paste. The cavity is sealed with a suitable lining, such as resin-modified glass-ionomer cement, and restored conventionally. The tooth should be carefully monitored.

Mineral trioxide aggregate

Although the majority of practitioners will use calcium hydroxide routinely and effectively for pulp capping and various repairs to the root, Mineral trioxide aggregate (MTA) is increasingly used in specialist and some general practices. The material is described briefly in Part 5, and the application discussed in Part 11. Early research as a root-end filling material showed unparalleled results, and workers have since reported similar success in other endodontic procedures, with no resulting inflammation, and deposition of cementum over the restorative material.[14–16] MTA can be used in place of hard-setting calcium hydroxide in all these pulp-capping procedures.

Root-end induction (apexification)

The cases in which partial or total closure of an open apex can be achieved are:

1. vital radicular pulp in an immature tooth pulpotomy (see Part 10);
2. pulpless immature tooth with or without a periapical radiolucent area.

Fig. 5 A calcific barrier is evident following calcium hydroxide therapy in a case with an open apex.

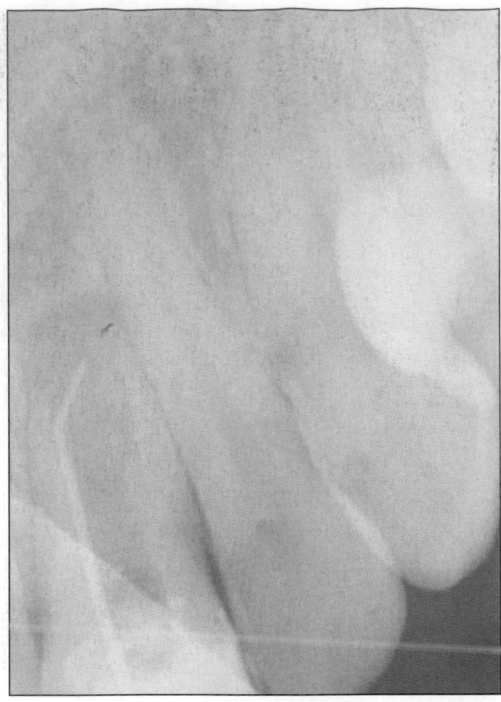

The success of closure is not related to the age of the patient. It is not possible to determine whether there would be continued root growth to form a normal root apex or merely the formation of a calcific barrier across the apical end of the root. The mode of healing would probably be related to the severity and duration of the periapical inflammation and the consequent survival of elements of Hertwig's sheath.

Inducing apical closure may take anything from 6 to 18 months or occasionally longer. It is necessary to change the calcium hydroxide during treatment; the suggested procedure is given below:

First visit – Thoroughly clean and prepare the root canal. Fill with calcium hydroxide.

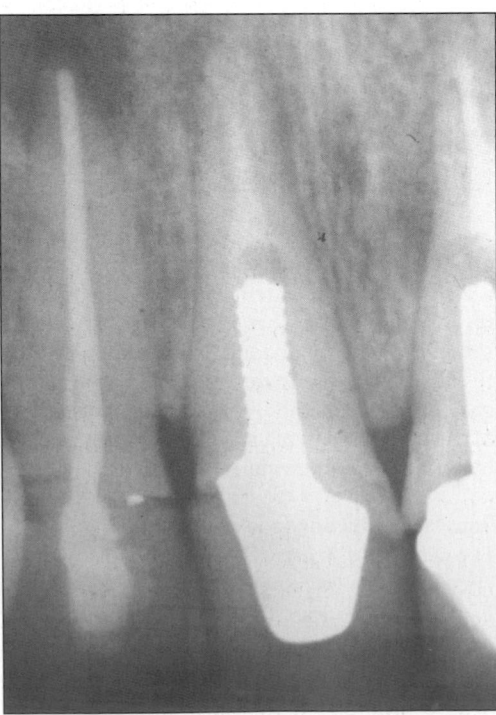

Fig. 6 The mesial wall of the root canal at tooth UL1 (21) has been perforated during post space preparation, causing a lateral periodontitis.

Second visit – 2 to 4 weeks later, remove the calcium hydroxide dressing with hand instruments and copious irrigation. Care should be taken not to disturb the periapical tissue. The root canal is dried and refilled with calcium hydroxide.

Third visit – 6 months later, a periapical radiograph is taken and root fill if closure is complete. This may be checked by removing the calcium hydroxide and tapping with a paper point against the barrier. Repeat the calcium hydroxide dressing if necessary.

Fourth visit – After a further 6 months another periapical radiograph is taken, and the tooth root-filled if closure is complete. If the barrier is still incomplete the calcium hydroxide dressing is repeated.

Fifth visit – This should take place 3 to 6 months later. The majority of root closures will have been completed by this time (Fig. 5).

Once again, however, reference must be made to the increasing use of MTA for root-end closure and other such endodontic procedures.[17]

Horizontal fractures

Horizontal fractures of the root may be treated, provided the fracture lies within the alveolar bone and does not communicate with the oral cavity. The blood supply may have been interrupted at the fracture site only, so that the apical fragment remains vital. In these cases, the coronal portion of the root can be treated as an open apex. Cvek states that healing with a calcific barrier can be achieved using calcium hydroxide.[15]

Iatrogenic perforations

Iatrogenic perforations are caused by an instrument breaching the apex or wall of the root canal; probably the most common occurrence is during the preparation of a post space (Fig. 6). Partial or complete closure by hard tissue may be induced with calcium hydroxide, provided the perforation is not too large, lies within the crestal bone and does not communicate with the oral cavity. Treatment should begin as soon as possible, adopting the same procedure as for root-end induction. Closure of perforations using calcium hydroxide takes considerably longer than root-end induction in most cases. An alternative technique, if the perforation can be visualized with the use of a surgical microscope, would be direct repair with mineral trioxide aggregate.

If foreign bodies in the form of root-filling materials, cements or separated instruments have been extruded into the tissues, healing with calcium hydroxide is unlikely to occur and a surgical approach is recommended (Part 11).

ROOT RESORPTION

Several different types of resorption are recognized: some are isolated to one tooth and slow spreading, others are rapid, aggressive and may involve several teeth. Resorption is initiated either from within the pulp, giving rise to

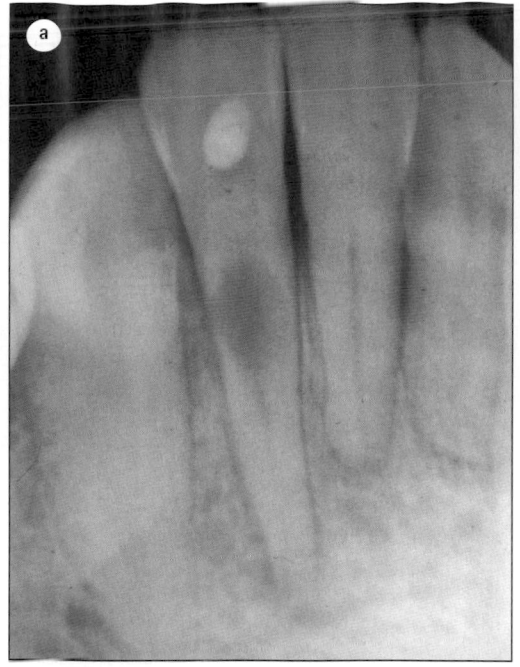 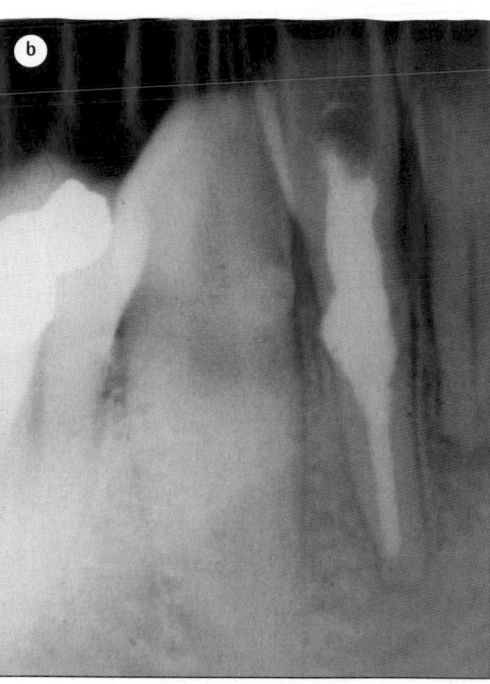

Fig. 7 a) Typical view of internal resorption, showing a smooth, rounded widening of the root canal. b) A warm gutta-percha technique will obturate the defect fully.

internal resorption, or from outside the tooth, where it is termed external resorption.

The aetiology of resorption has been described by Tronstad who also presented a new classification.[18] In Tronstad's view, the permanent teeth are not normally resorbed, the mineralized tissues are protected by predentine and odontoblasts in the root canal and by precementum and cementoblasts on the root surface. If the predentine or precementum becomes mineralized, or, in the case of the precementum, is mechanically damaged or scraped off, multinucleated cells colonize the mineralized or denuded surfaces and resorption ensues. Tronstad refers to this type of resorption as inflammatory, which may be transient or progressive. Transient inflammatory resorption will repair with the formation of a cementum-like tissue, unless there is continuous stimulation. Transient root resorption will occur in traumatized teeth or teeth that have undergone periodontal treatment or orthodontics. Progressive resorption may occur in the presence of infection, certain systemic diseases, mechanical irritation of tissue or increased pressure in tissue.

Internal resorption

The aetiology of internal resorption is thought to be the result of a chronic pulpitis. Tronstad believes that there must be a presence of necrotic tissue in order for internal resorption to become progressive.[18] In most cases, the condition is pain-free and so tends to be diagnosed during routine radiographic examination. Chronic pulpitis may follow trauma, caries or iatrogenic procedures such as tooth preparation, or the cause may be unknown. Internal resorption occurs infrequently, but may appear in any tooth; the tooth may be restored or caries-free. The defect may be located anywhere within the root canal system. When it occurs within the pulp chamber, it has been referred to as 'pink spot' because the

enlarged pulp is visible through the crown. The typical radiographic appearance is of a smooth and rounded widening of the walls of the root canal. If untreated, the lesion is progressive and will eventually perforate the wall of the root, when the pulp will become non-vital (Fig. 7a). The destruction of dentine may be so severe that the tooth fractures.

The treatment for non-perforated internal resorption is to extirpate the pulp and prepare and obturate the root canal. An inter-appointment dressing of calcium hydroxide may be used and a warm gutta-percha filling technique helps to obturate the defect (Fig. 7b). The main problem is the removal of the entire pulpal contents from the area of resorption while keeping the access to a minimum. Hand instrumentation using copious amounts of sodium hypochlorite is recommended. The ultrasonic technique of root canal preparation may provide a cleaner canal as the acoustic streaming effect removes canal debris from areas inaccessible to the file. The prognosis for these teeth is good and the resorption should not recur.

The treatment of internal resorption that has perforated is more difficult, as the defect must be sealed. When the perforation is inaccessible to a surgical approach, an intracanal seal may be achieved with a warm gutta-percha technique. Alternatively, the root canal and resorbed area may be obturated using mineral trioxide aggregate. Before the final root filling is placed, a calcium hydroxide dressing is recommended.

External resorption

There are many causes of external resorption, both general and local.[19] An alteration of the delicate balance between osteoblastic and osteoclastic action in the periodontal ligament will produce either a build-up of cementum on the root surface (hypercementosis) or its removal together with dentine, which is external resorption.

Fig. 8 a) Inflammatory resorption following periodontal treatment of a tooth with a necrotic pulp. b) Root canal treatment has been carried out, and the lesion repaired by a surgical approach.

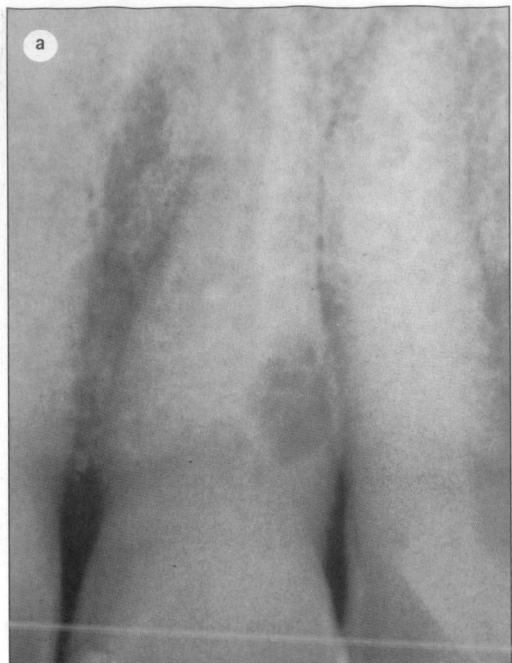
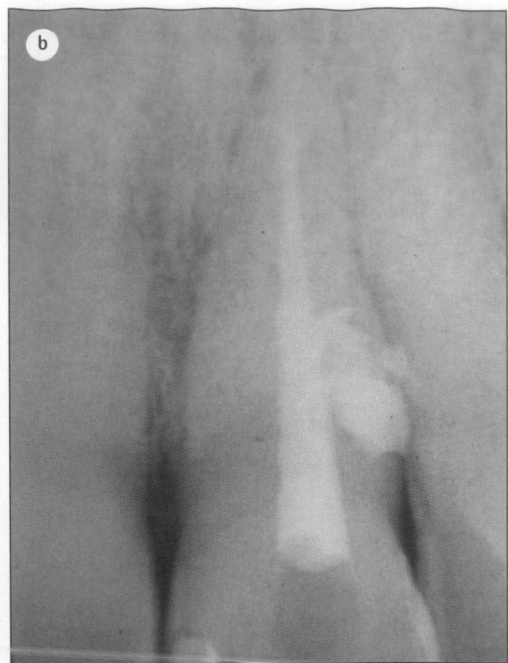

Resorption may be preceded by an increase in blood supply to an area adjacent to the root surface. The inflammatory process may be due to infection or tissue damage in the periodontal ligament, or, alternatively post-traumatic hyperplastic gingivitis and cases of epulis. It has been suggested that osteoclasts are derived from blood-borne monocytes. Inflammation increases the permeability of the associated capillary vessels, allowing the release of monocytes which then migrate towards the injured bone and/or root surface. Other causes of resorption include pressure, chemical, systemic diseases and endocrine disturbances.

Six different types of external resorption have been recognized and recorded in the literature.

Surface resorption
Surface resorption is a common pathological finding.[20] The condition is self-limiting and undergoes spontaneous repair. The root surface shows both superficial resorption lacunae and repair with new cementum. The osteoclastic activity is a response to localized injury to the periodontal ligament or cementum. Surface resorption is rarely evident on the radiograph.

Inflammatory resorption
Inflammatory resorption is thought to be caused by infected pulp tissue. The areas affected will be around the main apical foramina and lateral canal openings. The cementum, dentine and adjacent periodontal tissues are involved, and a radiolucent area is visible radiographically. In the case illustrated in Figure 8 the root canal was sclerosed following trauma at an early age. Root planing during periodontal treatment which removed the cementum layer appeared to be the initiating factor for inflammatory resorption around a lateral canal. The root canal was identified and root canal treatment carried out, followed by external surgical repair of the lesion.

Replacement resorption
Replacement resorption is a direct result of trauma and has been described in detail by Andreasen.[21] A high incidence of replacement resorption follows replantation and luxation, particularly if there was delay in replacing the tooth or there was an accompanying fracture of the alveolus. The condition has also been referred to as ankylosis, because there is gradual resorption of the root, accompanied by the simultaneous replacement by bony trabeculae. Radiographically, the periodontal ligament space will be absent, the bone merging imperceptibly with the dentine.

Once started, this condition is usually irreversible, leading ultimately to the replacement of the entire root. Calcium hydroxide treatment is unlikely to help in the treatment of this type of resorption.

Pressure resorption
Pressure on a tooth can eventually cause resorption provided there is a layer of connective tissue between the two surfaces. Pressure can be caused by erupting or impacted teeth, orthodontic movement, trauma from occlusion, or pathological tissue such as a cyst or neoplasm. Resorption due to orthodontic treatment is relatively common. One report of a 5–10-year follow-up after completion of orthodontic treatment found an incidence of 28.8% of affected incisors.[22]

It may be assumed that the pressure exerted evokes a release of monocyte cells and the subsequent formation of osteoclasts. If the cause of the pressure is removed, the resorption will be arrested.

Systemic resorption
This may occur in a number of systemic diseases and endocrine disturbances: hyperparathyroidism, Paget's disease, calcinosis, Gaucher's disease and Turner's syndrome. In addition,

resorption may occur in patients following radiation therapy.

Idiopathic resorption

There are many reports of cases in which, despite investigation, no possible local or general cause has been found. The resorption may be confined no one tooth, or several may be involved. The rate of resorption varies from slow, taking place over years, to quick and aggressive, involving large amounts of tissue destruction over a few months. The site and shape of the resorption defect also varies. Two different types of idiopathic resorption have been described.

Apical resorption is usually slow and may arrest spontaneously; one or several teeth may be affected, with a gradual shortening of the root, while the root apex remains rounded. Cervical external resorption takes place in the cervical area of the tooth. The defect may form either a wide, shallow crater or, conversely, a burrowing type of resorption. This latter type has been described variously as peripheral cervical resorption, burrowing resorption, pseudo pink spot, resorption extra camerale and extracanal invasive.

There is a small defect on the external surface of the tooth; the resorption then burrows deep into the dentine with extensive tunnel-shaped ramifications. It does not, as a rule, affect the dentine and predentine in the immediate vicinity of the pulp. This type of resorption is easily mistaken for internal resorption. Cervical resorption may be caused by chronic inflammation of the periodontal ligament or by trauma. Both types of cervical resorption are best treated by surgical exposure of the resorption lacunae and removal of the granulation tissue. The resorptive defect is then shaped to receive a restoration.

THE PERIO-ENDO LESION

The differential diagnosis of perio-endo lesions has become increasingly important as the demand for complicated restorative work has grown. Neither periodontic nor endodontic treatment can be considered in isolation as clinically they are closely related and this must influence the diagnosis and treatment. The influence of infected and necrotic pulp on the periapical tissues is well known, but there remains much controversy over the effect that periodontal disease could have on a vital pulp.

Examination of the anatomy of the tooth shows that there are many paths to be taken by bacteria and their toxic products between the pulp and the periodontal ligament. Apart from the main apical foramina, lateral canals exist in approximately 50% of teeth, and may be found in the furcation region of permanent molars.[23] Seltzer *et al.* observed inter-radicular periodontal changes in dogs and monkeys after inducing pulpotomies and concluded that noxious material passed through dentinal tubules in the floor of the pulp chamber.[24] In addition to dentinal tubules, microfractures are often present in teeth, allowing the passage of microorganisms. Clinically, it is common to see cervical sensitivity.

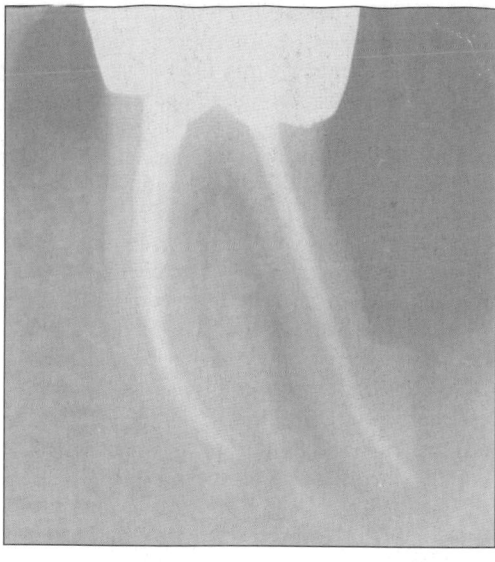

Fig. 9 A severe endo-perio lesion that may require root resection.

The controversy concerning the effect of periodontal disease on the pulp ranges between those who believe that pulpitis or pulp necrosis or both can occur as a result of periodontal inflammation, to those who state categorically that pulpal changes are independent of the status of the periodontium. In the author's opinion, Belk and Gutmann present the most rational view, which is that periodontal disease may damage pulp tissue via accessory or lateral canals, but total pulpal disintegration will not occur unless all the main apical foramina are involved by bacterial plaque (Fig. 9).[25]

The problem that faces the clinician treating perio-endo lesions is to assess the extent of the disease and to decide whether the tooth or the periodontium is the primary cause. Only by carrying out a careful examination can the operator judge the prognosis and plan the treatment.[26] There are several ways in which perio-endo lesions can be classified; the one given below is a slight modification of the Simon, Glick and Frank classification.[27]

Classification of perio-endo lesions

Class 1. Primary endodontic lesion draining through the periodontal ligament

Class 1 lesions present as an isolated periodontal pocket or swelling beside the tooth. The patient rarely complains of pain, although there will often be a history of an acute episode. The cause of the pocket is a necrotic pulp draining through the periodontal ligament. The furcation area of both premolar and molar teeth may be involved. Diagnostically, one should suspect a pulpally induced lesion when the crestal bone levels on both the mesial and distal aspects appear normal and only the furcation shows a radiolucent area.

Class 2. Primary endodontic lesion with secondary periodontal involvement

If left untreated, the primary lesion may become secondarily involved with periodontal breakdown. A probe may encounter plaque or calculus in the pocket. The lesion will resolve partially with root canal treatment but complete repair will involve periodontal therapy.

Class 3. Primary periodontal lesions

Class 3 lesions are caused by periodontal disease gradually spreading along the root surface. The pulp, although compromised, may remain vital. However, in time there will be degenerative changes. The tooth may become mobile as the attachment apparatus and surrounding bone are destroyed, leaving deep periodontal pocketing. Perodontal disease will usually be seen elsewhere in the mouth unless there are local predisposing factors such as a severely defective restoration or proximal groove.

Class 4. Primary periodontal lesions with secondary endodontic involvement

A Class 3 lesion progresses to a Class 4 lesion with the involvement of the main apical foramina or possibly a large lateral canal. It is sometimes difficult to decide whether the lesion is primarily endodontic with secondary periodontal involvement (Class 2), or primarily periodontal with secondary endodontic involvement (Class 4), particularly in the late stages. If there is any doubt, the necrotic pulp should be removed; any improvement in the periodontal disease suggests that the classification was in fact of a Class 2 lesion.

Root removal and root canal treatment

To prevent further destruction of the periodontium in multirooted teeth, in may be necessary to remove one or occasionally two roots. As this treatment will involve root canal therapy and periodontal surgery, the operator must consider the more obvious course of treatment, which is to extract the tooth and provide some form of fixed prosthesis. As a guide, the following factors should be considered before root resection:

1 *Functional tooth.* The tooth should be a functional member of the dentition.
2 *Root filling.* It should be possible to provide root canal treatment which has a good prognosis. In other words, the root canals must be fully negotiable.
3 *Anatomy.* The roots should be separate with some inter-radicular bone so that the removal of one root will not damage the remaining root(s). Access to the tooth must be sufficient to allow the correct angulation of the handpiece to remove the root. A small mouth may contra-indicate the procedure.
4 *Restorable.* Sufficient tooth structure must remain to allow the tooth to be restored. The finishing line of the restoration must be envisaged to ensure that it will be cleansable by the patient.
5 *Patient suitability.* The patient must be a suitable candidate for the lengthy operative procedures and be able to maintain a high standard of oral cleanliness around the sectioned tooth.

A tooth that requires a root to be resected will need root canal treatment. The surgery must be planned with care, particularly with respect to the timing of the root treatment. Ideally, the tooth should be root filled prior to surgery, except for the root to be resected. The pulp is extirpated from the root to be removed, the canal widened in the coronal 2–3 mm and restored with a permanent material. This means a retrograde filling will not have to be placed at the time of surgery – a procedure which is difficult to perform owing to poor access and blood contamination of the filling and the likelihood of the restorative material falling into the socket.

1. Hermann B W. Dentinobleration der Wurzelkanale nach der Behandlung mit Kalcium. *Zahnarzt Rundschau* 1930; **39**: 888.
2. Sciaky I, Pisanti S. Localisation of calcium placed over amputated pulps in dogs' teeth. *J Dent Res* 1960; **39**: 1128–1132.
3. Tronstad L, Andreason J O, Hasselgren G, Kristerson L, Riis I. PH changes in dental tissues after root canal filling with calcium hydroxide. *J Endod* 1981; **7**: 17–21.
4. Hasselgren G, Tronstad L. Enzyme activity in the pulp following preparation of cavities and insertion of medicaments in cavities in monkeys. *Acta Odontol Scand* 1978; **35**: 289–295.
5. Tronstad L, Mjør I A. Pulp reactions to calcium hydroxide containing materials *Oral Surgery, Oral Medicine, Oral Pathology* 1972; **33**: 961–965
6. Bergenholtz G, Reit C. Reactions of the dental pulp to microbial provocation of calcium hydroxide treated dentine. *Scand J Dent Res* 1980; **88**: 187–192.
7. Warfvinge J, Rozell B, Hedström K G. Effect of calcium hydroxide treated dentine on pulpal responses. *Int Endod J* 1987; **20**: 183–193.
8. Kidd E A M, Banerjee A. What is Absence of Caries. In Albrektsson TO, Bratthall D, Glantz P-O J and Lindhe JT, *Tissue Preservation in Caries Treatment.* London: Quintessence Books, 2001.
9. Kim S, Trowbridge H, Suda H. Chapter 15 in Cohen S and Burns R C, *Pathways of the Pulp Eighth* Edition. St Louis: Mosby, 2002.
10. Hasselgren G. Chapter 9 in Ørstavik D and Pitt Ford T R. *Essential Endodontology* Oxford: Blackwell Science, 1998.
11. Kakehashi S, Stanley H R, Fitzgerald R J. The effects of surgical exposures of dental pulps in germ-free and conventional laboratory rats. *Oral Surgery, Oral Medicine, Oral Pathology* 1965; **20**: 340–349.
12. Cvek M. A clinical report on partial pulpotomy and capping with calcium hydroxide in permanent incisors with complicated crown fracture. *J Endod* 1978; **4**: 232–237.
13. Fuks A B, Chosack A, Klein H, Eidelman E. Partial pulpotomy as a treatment alternative for exposed pulps in crown-fractured permanent incisors. *Endod Dent Traumatol* 1987; **3**: 10–102.
14. Torabinejad M, Hong C U, Lee S J, Monsef M, Pitt Ford T R. Investigation of mineral trioxide aggregate for root-end filling in dogs. *J Endod* 1995; **21**: 603–608.
15. Schwartz R S, Mauger M, Clement D J, Walker W A. Mineral trioxide aggregate: a new material for endodontics. *J Am Dent Assoc* 1999; **130**: 967–975.
16. Witherspoon D E, Ham K. One-visit apexification: technique for inducing root end barrier formation in apical closures. *Practical Proceedings in Aesthetic Dentistry* 2001; **13**: 455–460.
17. Cvek M. Treatment of non-vital permanent incisors with calcium hydroxide IV. Periodontal healing and closure of the root canal in the coronal fragment of teeth with intra-alveolar fracture and vital apical fragment. A follow-up. *Odont Revy* 1974; **25**: 239–246.
18. Tronstad L. Root resorption – aetiology, terminology and clinical manifestations. *Endod Dent Traumatol* 1988; **4**: 241–252.
19. Newman W G. Possible etiologic factors in external root resorption. *Am J Orthod* 1975; **67**: 522–539.
20. Henry J L, Weinmann J P. The pattern of resorption and repair of human cementum. *J Am Dent Assoc* 1951; **42**: 270–290.

21. Andreasen J O. *Textbook and Colour Atlas of Traumatic Injuries of the Teeth*. Denmark: Munksgaard, 1993.

22. Cwyk F, Scat-Pierre F Tronstad L. Endodontic implications of orthodontic tooth movement. *J Dent Res* 1984; **63**: Abstract 1039.

23. Gutmann J L. Prevalence, location and frequency of accessory canals in the furcation region of permanent molars. *J Periodontol* 1978; **49**: 21–26.

24. Seltzer S, Bender I B, Nazimor M, Sinai I. Pulpitis-induced inter-radicular periodontal changes in experimental animals. *J Periodontol* 1967; **38**: 124–129.

25. Belk C E, Gutmann J L. Perspectives, controversies and directives on pulpal-periodontal relationships. *J Can Dent Assoc* 1990; **56**: 1013–1017.

26. Solomon C, Chalfin H, Kellert M, Weseley P. The endodontic-periodontal lesion: a rational approach to treatment. *J Am Dent Assoc* 1995; **126**: 473–479.

27. Simon J H, Glick D H, Frank A L. The relationship of endodontic-periodontic lesions. *J Periodontol* 1972; **43**: 202–208.

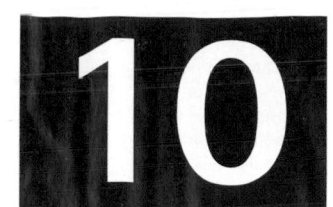

IN BRIEF

- Root canal treatment in children should only be prescribed after careful consideration of the patient, the existing dentition, and developing teeth.
- Isolation with rubber dam is just as important as with the permanent dentition.
- Paediatric endodontic treatment may be more directed towards pulpotomy rather than pulpectomy.
- All practitioners should be familiar with current guidelines on the treatment of the avulsed tooth.

Endodontic treatment for children

Root canal treatment for children has particular difficulties and considerations. It must be planned in light of the remaining teeth, and the need for balancing or compensating extraction borne in mind. Diagnosis may be difficult, as may prolonged treatment under local anaesthesia and rubber dam. Vital pulpotomy techniques with formocresol and/or calcium hydroxide must be carefully executed in line with the UK National Guidelines. The treatment of the avulsed tooth has been the subject of much research, and practitioners should ensure that they are up-to-date with current treatment modalities.

Although the basic aims of endodontic therapy in children are the same as those in adults, ie the removal of infection and chronic inflammation and thus the relief of associated pain, there are particular difficulties and considerations. The pulpal tissue of primary teeth may become involved far earlier in the advancing carious lesion than in permanent teeth. Exposure may also occur far more frequently during cavity preparation due to the enamel and dentine being thinner than in the permanent tooth, and the pulp chamber, with its extended pulp horns, being relatively larger, as can be seen in the extracted tooth at Figure 1. Primary molar root canals are irregular and ribbon-like in shape. Periradicular lesions associated with infected primary molars are usually inter-radicular

(Fig. 2) rather than periapical in site due to the presence of accessory canals in the thin floor of the pulp chamber.

As well as the problems associated with the primary dentition, endodontic treatment of permanent teeth in children may also present difficulties due to the incomplete root development and associated open apices.

BALANCED EXTRACTIONS

Primary teeth with pulpal exposure or pathology must always be treated, either by root canal treatment or by extraction. The maintenance of arch length is important for good masticatory function and the future eruption of the permanent dentition with optimal development of the occlusion. Whilst it is preferable to conserve a

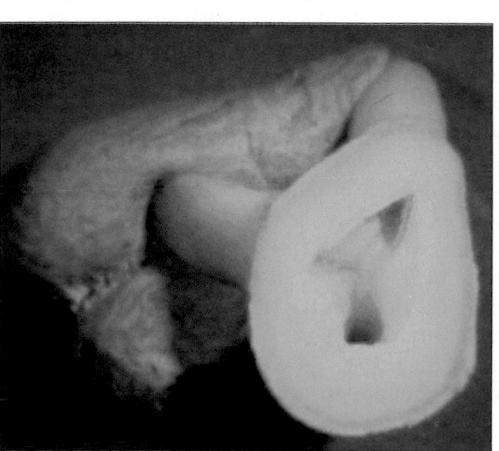

Fig. 1 An extracted deciduous molar showing the relatively large pulp chamber and root canals.

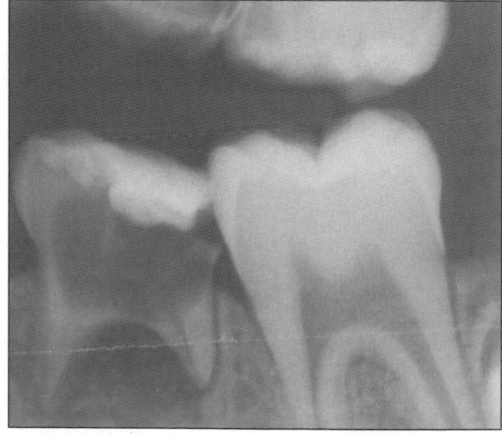

Fig. 2 A radiograph of a grossly carious lower second primary molar showing interadicular bone loss.

Fig. 3 A dental panoramic tomograph taken as part of the assessment for extraction of deciduous molars, reveals the absence of permanent lower second premolars.

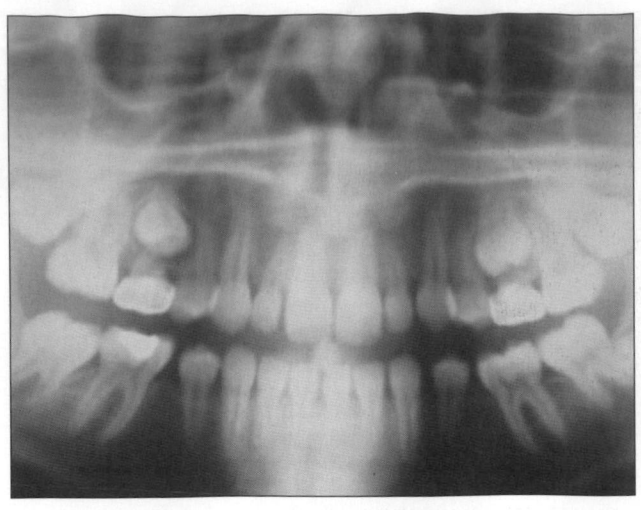

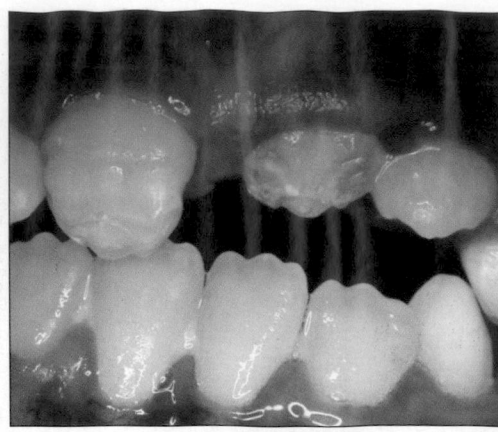

Fig. 4 Enamel hypoplasia of an upper permanent incisor following infection of the primary predecessor.

tooth rather than carry out an extraction, if this does become necessary, balanced extractions should always be kept in mind. A *balanced extraction* is the removal of a tooth from the opposite side of the same arch. A *compensating* extraction, removing a tooth from the opposing arch to the enforced extraction is more difficult to justify.[1] Balanced extractions are rarely justified for primary incisors. The loss of a primary canine, however, may have a significant effect on the arch and balanced extractions should always be considered. When a primary molar has to be extracted it may be preferable to prevent drifting with a space maintainer than carry out balanced extractions.

Extractions should be avoided wherever possible in certain groups of children; ie those with bleeding disorders, or medical conditions such as diabetes where general anaesthesia is contra-indicated. Primary teeth should also be retained where a radiograph reveals the lack of a permanent successor, as in Figure 3, where the patient may find pulp therapy less stressful than extraction, and in an already crowded dentition where tooth loss would lead to even further crowding of the permanent teeth.

ENDODONTIC TREATMENT OF PRIMARY TEETH

Endodontic treatment may be indicated far earlier when treating the primary dentition than in permanent teeth. Obviously, treatment is indicated when a patient presents with a pulpal necrosis, or symptoms of pulpitis. However, the distinction of reversible or irreversible pulpitis applied to the permanent teeth is not so relevant in the primary teeth; any sign or symptom of pulpitis indicates the need for pulp therapy. Current research and practice also suggests that pulp therapy will be necessary when a radiograph shows a carious lesion extending more than halfway through the dentine, or where the carious process has led to the loss of the marginal ridge.

However, there are important assessments to be made as to the patient's suitability for endodontic treatment. The general health of the patient should be checked to ensure that there are no contra-indications to endodontic therapy,

such as those with congenital heart disease, or patients who are immunocompromised. The attitude of the parent to treatment and the child's ability to cooperate during the more lengthy procedures require careful evaluation. The overall dental health of the child, with particular reference to the caries experience, must be taken into account when making a treatment plan. In a poorly cared for dentition requiring multiple treatments, the complex conservation of one tooth in the presence of a number of comparable teeth of doubtful prognosis is poor paediatric dentistry and should be avoided. In addition, root canal treatment should be avoided in grossly decayed teeth which may be unrestorable even after pulp therapy; in teeth where caries has penetrated the floor of the pulp chamber; in teeth with advanced root resorption, or those close to exfoliation.

An additional problem is the close relationship of the roots of the primary teeth to the developing permanent successor. During exfoliation, the roots of the former resorb, necessitating the use of a resorbable paste in endodontic treatment. It is also important to remember that trauma to, or infection of, a primary tooth, may result in damage to the permanent tooth. This may vary from enamel hypomineralization and hypoplasia to, more rarely, the delayed or arrested development of the tooth germ (Fig. 4).

Diagnosis

The reaction of pulp tissue in primary teeth to deep caries differs from that seen in the permanent dentition and is characterized by the rapid spread of inflammatory changes throughout the coronal portion of the tooth. These pathological changes become irreversible and, if left untreated, will involve the radicular tissue. There may be few, if any, clinical symptoms in the early stages to indicate the extent of tissue damage. Pain may only occur after involvement of the periradicular tissues in the spread of infection.

Children are often unable to give accurate details of their symptoms, and the responses to clinical tests may be unreliable. Difficulties are frequently experienced in ascertaining the condition of the pulp from clinical findings.

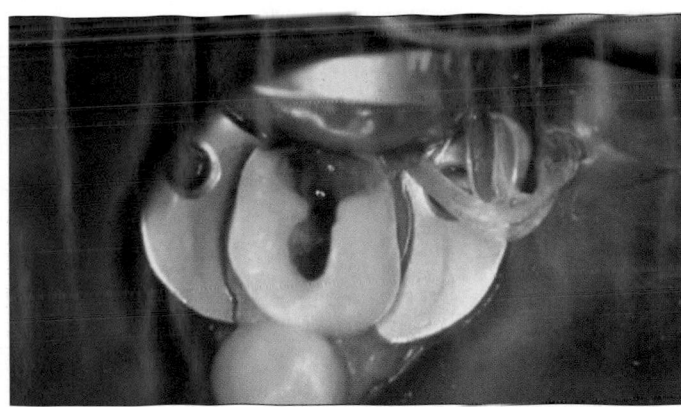

Fig. 5 A deciduous molar with a deep carious lesion has been isolated prior to commencing endodontic therapy.

Radiographs, which are essential prior to the commencement of treatment, may give little information of early pathological changes.

Before commencing treatment

The majority of the following restorative procedures will require adequate local anaesthesia. In accordance with the biological principles established throughout this text, adequate isolation will also be necessary to prevent salivary contamination. A rubber dam should be placed, and isolation completed with cotton wool rolls and saliva ejector as seen in Figure 5.

Indirect pulp capping

The aim of this treatment is to maintain the vitality of the pulp in a deep carious lesion, when there is no direct pulpal involvement. All the carious dentine must be removed, and a thin layer of sound, non-carious dentine must remain. A lining of setting calcium hydroxide is placed, which stimulates the formation of secondary dentine. The tooth is restored over the dressing with a permanent restorative material.

It has been suggested that other medicaments may be used for indirect pulp caps, for example antibiotic pastes and anti-inflammatory drugs, but although some success has been reported, pulp necrosis and abscess formation often result without symptoms. As with the permanent dentition, research is presently focussing on the use of adhesive materials and bonding agents for indirect pulp capping. The long-term results of these long-term clinical trials are awaited.

It should be noted that one technique for indirect pulp capping, which was described in the past, is no longer recommended. This was where deep caries was carefully excavated, avoiding pulpal exposure, and the deeper layers of softened dentine dressed with a calcium hydroxide-containing cement and a long-term temporary dressing. After a period of 6–8 weeks the tooth, which should have been symptomless, was reopened, and the arrested carious lesion examined. The success of this treatment was found to be less predictable and symptoms frequently developed. It is now recommended that all caries be removed, and if a pulpal exposure is found then either a direct pulp cap or a form of pulpotomy is used.

Direct pulp capping

This treatment is only recommended when a small traumatic exposure occurs, during cavity preparation of a vital non-infected pulp.[2] A calcium hydroxide dressing is placed directly over the pulp, followed by a lining and restoration, and the whole technique is carried out using local anaesthesia and with adequate isolation from salivary contamination. It has been suggested that the high cellular content of primary pulp tissue may be responsible for the failure of direct pulp capping in primary teeth.[3] Undifferentiated mesenchymal cells may differentiate into osteoclastic cells in response to either the caries or direct pulp capping which leads to internal resorption. It is also suggested that exposures on axial walls have a poor prognosis as the pulp coronal to the exposure may be deprived of its blood supply and undergo necrosis.

Vital pulpotomy techniques

These techniques involve the removal of inflamed coronal pulp tissue and the application of a dressing to the radicular pulp in an attempt to either promote healing of, or fix, the upper portions, and to preserve the vitality of the apical tissue. Because of the difficulties involved in diagnosing the condition of the pulp tissue histologically before the commencement of treatment, careful assessment must be made at each stage of the procedure. Whenever the haemorrhage from the radicular pulp stumps is profuse and uncontrolled, the assumption is made that the inflammatory process has extended into the radicular tissue, and the therapy modified accordingly. There are three pulpotomy techniques.

Vital formocresol pulpotomy

The treatment is carried out using local anaesthesia and adequate isolation. Following cavity preparation in the normal manner, the deep caries is removed and the coronal pulp chamber opened, such that there is no overhanging dentine inhibiting the complete removal of the pulp tissue. The coronal tissue is removed using a large excavator or sterile rosehead bur. If a high-speed diamond bur is used it should be cooled with sterile water or saline. Sterile cotton wool is applied to the radicular pulp tissue to achieve haemostasis. A small pledget of cotton wool is dipped in a 1:5 dilution of Buckley's formocresol (Table 1) and

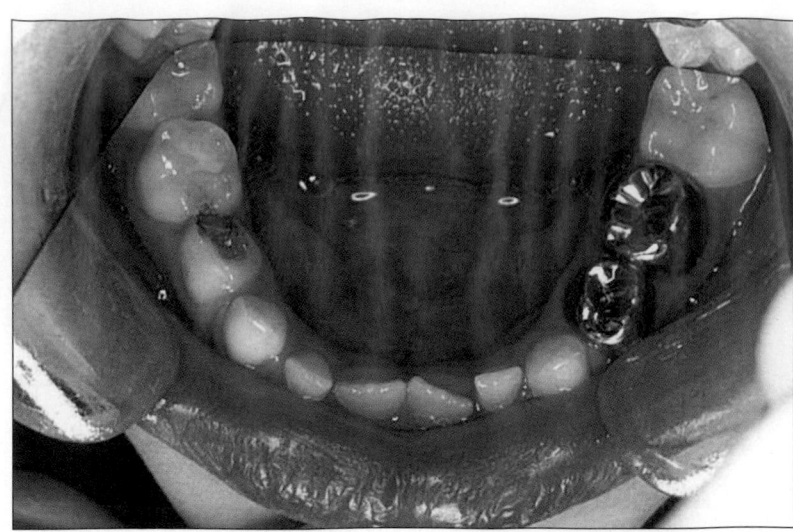

Fig. 6 Stainless steel crowns make ideal restorations for compromised deciduous molars.

Table 1 Buckley's formocresol	
Tricresol	35%
Formaldehyde	19%
Glycerol	15%
Water	31%

Table 2 Paraformaldehyde devitalizing paste	
Paraformaldehyde	1.00 g
Carbowax 1500	1.30 g
Lignocaine	0.06 g
Propylene glycol	0.5 ml
Carmine	10 mg

squeezed to remove excess liquid. It is placed over the radicular pulp stump for 5 minutes in order to fix the inflamed tissue and bacteria and thus allow healing of the unaffected pulp. If the haemorrhage has completely stopped, a layer of zinc oxide–eugenol or glass-ionomer cement is applied, and the tooth restored, preferably with a preformed stainless steel crown to prevent subsequent fracture of the weakened tooth (Fig. 6).

Other materials have been considered as an alternative to formocresol.[4] Concerns about the safety of formocresol led to investigations of pulpotomies employing a 2% glutaraldehyde solution as an alternative dressing, but research has shown a lower clinical success rate than with formocresol. Concern about hypersensitivity to and handling of glutaraldehyde have largely led to its abandonment as a treatment alternative.

Recent work by Waterhouse *at al.* has shown that very favourable results have been achieved with calcium hydroxide when it has been applied in carefully controlled circumstances.[5] Following haemostasis, calcium hydroxide powder was delivered to the pulp chamber using a small, sterile, endodontic amalgam carrier. The powder is condensed over the pulp stumps with an amalgam condensor and small pledgets of cotton wool. Failure of this technique is explained by the presence of an extra-pulpal clot separating the calcium hydroxide from the pulpal tissue and thus impairing healing.[3]

Both the calcium content and alkaline properties of the dressing are important to achieve healing. An initial layer of necrotic tissue develops, which becomes associated with an inflammatory reaction. Subsequently, a matrix forms and mineralizes to become a hard tissue barrier of dentine like-material.

Devitalization pulpotomy

This is a two-stage procedure, used when local anaesthesia cannot be obtained to permit extirpation of the pulp, or when haemorrhage is uncontrolled before or following the application of formocresol. This technique mummifies and fixes the coronal pulp tissue, whilst the major part of the radicular pulp remains vital, but it carries a lower success rate.[6]

If the tooth is not anaesthetized, cavity preparation is carried out as far as possible and access is gained to the pulpal exposure. A small amount of paraformaldehyde devitalizing paste (Table 2) on a pledget of cotton wool is applied to the exposed pulp tissue. Formaldehyde vapour liberated from the dressing permeates through the pulpal space, producing fixation of the tissues. A soft layer of zinc oxide–eugenol temporary dressing is then placed, without applying pressure, to seal the medicament in position. The child and parent must be warned of possible discomfort, for which analgesics are recommended. After one to two weeks the tooth is checked for signs and symptoms. The devitalized coronal pulp may now be removed, without the need for local anaesthesia. A hard setting layer of zinc oxide–eugenol, which may be mixed with formocresol, is then placed over the radicular stumps and the tooth restored. If some vital tissue remains in the coronal pulp chamber, a further dressing of paraformaldehyde paste is required.

Non-vital pulpotomy

This technique has been advocated where there is irreversible change in the radicular pulp, or where the pulp is completely non-vital, but where pulpectomy and root canal treatment is considered impractical. The little clinical evidence available suggests a limited prognosis of approximately 50%. At the first visit the necrotic pulp contents are removed as before, and, using small excavators, as much as possible of the radicular tissue. Beechwood creosote solution (Table 3) on a cotton pledget is sealed into the cavity with a zinc oxide–eugenol dressing.

One to two weeks later the tooth is checked for signs and symptoms. If there is evidence of infection (sinus, pain, swelling or mobility) a further beechwood creosote dressing should be placed. If, however, symptoms have resolved, the tooth may be restored as with the previous pulpotomy techniques.

Pulpectomy

Pulpectomy is indicated where the pulp is either non-vital or irreversibly inflamed. Although the technique is often considered difficult because of the complexity of the root canals in primary molars, clinical studies have shown a reasonably prognosis.[7] The cavity preparation and removal of the necrotic coronal pulp is carried out as previously described. If the radicular pulp is necrotic, a two-stage procedure is required, but if it is found to be irreversibly inflamed a one-stage technique may be undertaken.

One-stage technique

The root canals are identified and instrumented to the working length estimated from a pre-operative radiograph. After drying the canals with paper points, formocresol is applied for up to 5 minutes. The root canals are then filled with a thin mix of zinc oxide–eugenol, using a rotary paste filler, and the restoration of the tooth is completed.

Two-stage technique

Here the root canals are again cleaned, shaped and irrigated to remove all necrotic debris. A pledget of cotton wool moistened with either formocresol or beechwood creosote is sealed in the pulp chamber with a rigid zinc oxide–eugenol dressing for one week. At the subsequent visit the tooth should be symptom-free, firm, without a discharging sinus. (If not, a second application of beechwood creosote is required.) If the tooth is found to be symptomless, a dressing of zinc oxide–eugenol, with or without the addition of formocresol, is packed into the base of the chamber and the tooth finally restored.

The preceding techniques are reviewed in the UK National Guidelines.[8]

Review

Following any form of endodontic treatment, regular clinical and radiographic reviews must be made of the tooth involved and its successor. If rarefaction of the bone in the furcation area is seen further pulpectomy may be possible, but extraction is probably indicated. Radiographs should also be checked for evidence of internal resorption, which may occur in limited areas in formocresol pulpotomies, but may be more extensive following the use of calcium hydroxide. It may progress to cause perforation of the

Table 3 Beechwood creosote	
0-Methoxy phenol (Guaicol)	47%
P-Methoxy phenol	26%
2-Methoxy, 4 methyl phenol (Cresol)	13%
M-Methoxy phenol	7%
Other	7%

root. Inflammatory follicular cysts[9] may develop, which necessitate the removal of the primary tooth and marsupialization of the cyst to allow the permanent tooth to erupt.

PERMANENT DENTITION
Immature permanent incisors

Although one in five children will suffer trauma to their developing permanent incisors, only about 6% of these will subsequently become non-vital and require endodontic treatment. The correct initial diagnosis of such traumatized teeth, based on signs and symptoms, radiographic examination and sensibility testing, is therefore very important. Laser Doppler flowmetry has shown that traumatized immature teeth with open apices may have a vital pulp even in the absence of a response to conventional sensibility testing. If there is any uncertainty about the vitality of the pulp, root canal treatment should be deferred and the tooth kept under regular review.

If, however, endodontic treatment of an immature permanent tooth with an open apex is indicated, a root-end closure technique is necessary to form a calcific barrier against which the obturation may eventually be compacted without extruding material into the periradicular tissues (Fig. 7).

The tooth should be isolated with rubber dam, and the pulp chamber accessed. Local anaesthesia is usually given as some vital tissue may still be encountered during pulp extirpation. In severe cases an intracanal steroid dressing, such as Ledermix, may be required for one week. Canal preparation is carried out with files to approximately 1–2 mm short of the working length, estimated from the pre-operative radiograph and confirmed during treatment. Copious irrigation with a sodium hypochlorite solution is necessary to remove all necrotic debris. The root canal should be dried with paper points, and then filled to the apex with calcium hydroxide paste, compressed with large paper points and/or cotton pledgets. The access cavity should be sealed with a long-term temporary dressing, such as glass-ionomer cement.

After one month, the dressing is carefully removed with copious irrigation, and the dried canal refilled with calcium hydroxide paste. After a further 3 to 6 months the tooth is opened again and a large paper point used at working length to feel for a calcific barrier. The paper point is gently inserted into the clean, dry canal. At the estimated working length either the point will remain dry, tap against a hard barrier, with

Fig. 7 a) An immature tooth with a non-vital pulp has been filled with calcium hydroxide b).

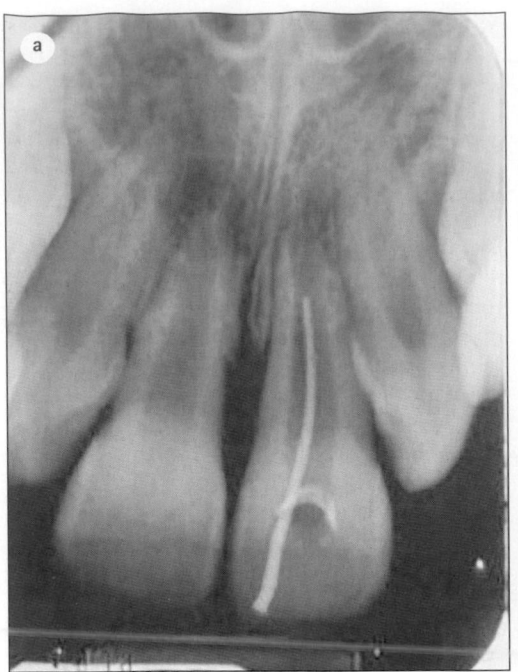
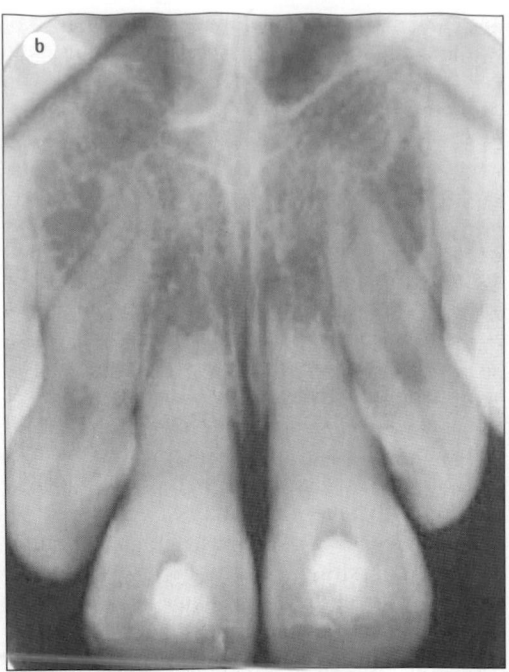

no sensation to the patient indicating closure, or will press against soft granulation tissue which the patient will feel. The average time taken for closure is 6 months.

If no barrier is detected, the calcium hydroxide is replaced. If the open apex is found to be completely closed the canal may be obturated with gutta-percha and sealer. Closure of an open apex may be anticipated in over 90% of cases treated by this technique, with a 4-year prognosis of 85%.[10] Obturation may then be completed by one of several methods. Conventional cold lateral compaction may be used, perhaps inverting a large gutta-percha point to obtain a good apical tug-back. A custom gutta-percha point may be made by rolling several GP points together after softening in solvent or gentle heat, and repeated fitting to the canal, carefully marking the orientation at insertion. However, injectable thermo-plasticized gutta-percha may be the most suitable obturation medium.

First permanent molar

The first permanent molar may, soon after eruption, show extensive caries, sometimes associated with hypoplasia. Consideration must be given to the age of the patient and the dental development, the occlusion and possible need for orthodontic treatment, as well as the long-term restorative prognosis of the tooth and the patient's ability to tolerate involved treatment over a long period. Where necessary, planned extractions should be considered. The primary aim of conservation is to ensure that root growth continues with completion of apical formation, so that definitive endodontic treatment, if required, may be carried out at a later stage.

The vitality of the tooth must be assessed and radiographs should be available, showing the extent of carious involvement and the state of the periapical tissues. It is essential that a local anaesthetic is administered and salivary control achieved by adequate isolation. Caries should be excavated and the tooth treated in accordance with conventional protocols. If a small exposure of a vital tooth occurs, either accidentally during cavity preparation or because of caries, and the surrounding tissue is healthy, a direct pulp cap with calcium hydroxide cement may be applied. A lining of glass-ionomer cement is then placed to seal the dentine tubules prior to the definitive restoration. If amalgam is used, a dentine bonding system should be considered to ensure complete sealing of the restoration.

If the exposure is large and the vitality of the radicular pulp is to be maintained to allow for root development, a pulpotomy may be carried out. Following the opening of the coronal pulp chamber and the removal of the pulp tissue, the area is irrigated and dried. Haemostasis of the radicular pulp should be observed prior to the application of calcium hydroxide cement or paste, and the provision of a permanent restoration. A calcific barrier should develop adjacent to the dressing, and root development continue in the presence of healthy pulp tissue.

If the pulp of a young, permanent molar is found to be non-vital, endodontic treatment should be undertaken only after careful assessment of the developing occlusion, the condition of the comparable teeth, the patient's ability to cooperate and the long-term prognosis of the tooth. If pulpal necrosis occurs prior to the complete development of the apex, the objective of treatment, as described earlier, is to encourage further deposition of calcified tissue in the apical region. Thorough preparation of the root canals is carried out, avoiding damage to the apical tissues and cells of Hertwig's root sheath. Calcium hydroxide is then applied as previously described. Definitive endodontic treatment is carried out when an apical barrier has formed and the tooth is then permanently restored. If symptoms arise in fully developed, young, permanent teeth, conventional orthograde root-filling with gutta-percha and sealer is indicated.

Avulsed permanent teeth

In the emergency management of an avulsed permanent tooth, time is of the essence. The long-term prognosis begins to deteriorate after only 15 minutes.[11] Most cases initially present with a telephone call. Where possible, re-implantation should be immediate, following rinsing if necessary in either milk (preferably) or tap water. The tooth should be held in place by biting gently on a soft cloth until splinting is possible by the dentist. If the person attending the accident is not prepared to re-implant the tooth, it should be stored in milk, normal saline or saliva (in the buccal sulcus) during the journey to the dental surgery.

Avoiding unnecessary delay, and keeping the tooth in the transport solution to prevent drying of the periodontal fibres, a thorough medical, dental and accident history should be taken and recorded. Local anaesthesia may be necessary to permit manipulation of the alveolar bone, and to enable gentle syringing of the socket with saline to remove any blood clot. The tooth, handled only by the crown, should be carefully inserted into the socket. Root canal treatment should NOT be commenced before re-implantation.

A non-rigid splint should be applied for 7–10 days, using acid-etched resin with a soft arch wire. The patient should be advised to avoid biting on the splinted tooth, take a soft diet, and maintain good oral hygiene with careful brushing and a chlorhexidine mouth-rinse. Systemic antibiotics may be indicated for medically compromised patients. The patient's tetanus status must be checked and a booster given by a medical practitioner if necessary. A review appointment should be made in 2 days to verify the splint, and modify it if necessary.

In very young patients where the tooth has a wide-open apex and was out of the mouth for only a short period there is a possibility of re-vascularization of the pulp. The tooth should be kept under almost weekly review, and if any clinical signs of non-vitality develop, such as tenderness, discoloration, swelling or sinus formation, endodontic treatment should be commenced immediately. Endodontic treatment should be commenced on all other avulsed teeth whilst the splint is in place. A long-term calcium hydroxide dressing should be sealed in place with a glass-ionomer restoration for at least 6 months prior to verification of an apical barrier and obturation as described earlier.

Replanted teeth should be regularly reviewed for at least 2–3 years, checking for inflammatory resorption, replacement resorption, ankylosis, infra-occlusion and discoloration. The adjacent teeth should also be reviewed. Resorption may commence within weeks of the injury.

Finally, it should be realized that there are some situations where replantation is not appropriate. For example:

- If the patient has other serious injuries, which should be given priority.
- If the patient has an at-risk medical history.
- Where the extra-oral time is very prolonged, the prognosis is very poor, particularly in teeth with short roots and wide apices.
- Primary teeth should not be replanted due to the possibility of damage to the permanent replacement.

ACKNOWLEDGEMENTS

Figures 1, 2, 3, 5, 6 and 7 have been reproduced by kind permission of Dr M-T Hosey, Children's Department, Glasgow University.

Figure 4 is reproduced by kind permission of Professor R R Welbury.

1. BSPD and IAPD. UK national guidelines in paediatric dentistry. *Int J Paediatr Dent* 2002; **12**: 151–153.
2. Kopel H M. Considerations for the direct pulp capping procedure in primary teeth: A review of the literature. *Paediatr Dent* 1992; **59**: 141–149.
3. Gould A, Johnstone S, Smith P. *Pulp Therapy techniques for the deciduous dentition.* (Compact Disk) London: King's College, 1999.
4. Waterhouse P J. Formocresol and alternative primary molar pulpotomy medicaments: a review. *Endod Dent Traumatol* 1991; **11**: 157–162.
5. Waterhouse P J, Nunn J H, Whitworth J M. An investigation of the relative efficacy of Buckley's Formocresol and Calcium Hydroxide in primary molar vital pulp therapy. *BDJ* 2000; **188**: 32–36.
6. Coll J A, Sadrian R. Predicting pulpotomy success and its relationship to exfoliation and succedaneous dentition. *Paediatr Dent* 1996; **18**: 57–63.
7. Barr E S, Flaitz C M, Hicks M J. A retrospective radiographic evaluation of primary molar pulpectomies. *Paediatr Dent* 2000; **13**: 4–9.
8. Llewelyn D R. UK national guidelines in paediatric dentistry. *Int J Paediatr Dent* 2000; **10**: 248–252.
9. Shaw W, Smith D M, Hill F J. Inflammatory follicular cysts. *J Dent Child* 1980; **47**: 97–101.
10. Mackie I C, Worthington H V, Hill F J. A follow up study of incisor teeth which have been treated by apical closure and root filling. *BDJ* 1993; **175**: 99–101.
11. Andersson L, Bodin I. Avulsed human teeth replanted within 15 minutes – a long term clinical follow-up study. *Endod Dent Traumatol* 1990; **6**: 37–42.

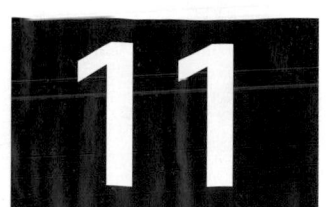

IN BRIEF

- A surgical approach to a failed root canal treatment should only be considered when an orthograde approach is not possible.
- The reason for failure should be carefully diagnosed before surgery is prescribed.
- Modern periradicular surgery involves the use of an operating microscope, microsurgical instruments, and appropriate retrograde sealing materials
- All surgical treatment should be followed-up, and encompassed in audit procedures.

Surgical endodontics

Root canal treatment usually fails because infection remains within the root canal. An orthograde attempt at re-treatment should always be considered first. However, when surgery is indicated, modern microtechniques coupled with surgical magnification will lead to a better prognosis. Careful management of the hard and soft tissues is essential, specially designed ultrasonic tips should be used for root end preparation which should ideally be sealed with MTA. All cases should be followed up until healing is seen, or failure accepted, and should form a part of clinical audit.

Although conventional orthograde root canal therapy must always be the preferred method of treating the diseased pulp, there are occasions when a surgical approach may be necessary. If orthograde treatment has failed to resolve the situation, the clinician should make every effort to ascertain why this has happened. A surgical approach is only indicated when it is agreed that orthograde retreatment is either not possible or will not solve the problem.

The two cases shown in Figures 1 and 2, both of which were referred for periradicular surgery, illustrate this point well. Figure 1 shows a radiograph of a lower molar that was causing symptoms, having first been obturated with silver

points and subsequently suffered surgery when the problem did not resolve. The correct treatment should have been a repeat of the orthograde treatment to remove the infection from within the root canal space that was causing the failure. Figure 2 shows totally inadequate endodontic treatment. The case requires total dismantling and thorough orthograde retreatment.

There have been considerable developments in periradicular surgery, both in technique and materials, in recent years.[1-6] Specialist practitioners routinely use surgical microscopes in conjunction with specially designed microsurgical instruments and retrograde filling materials. A description of these techniques is included in this chapter, and general practitioners are encouraged to compare this with their current practice, and adopt as many of these new

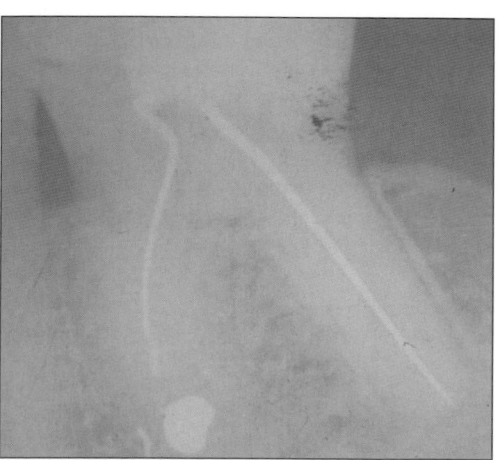

Fig. 1 This tooth has been obturated with silver points, and subsequently received periradicular surgery. The correct treatment should have been orthograde retreatment and conventional obturation.

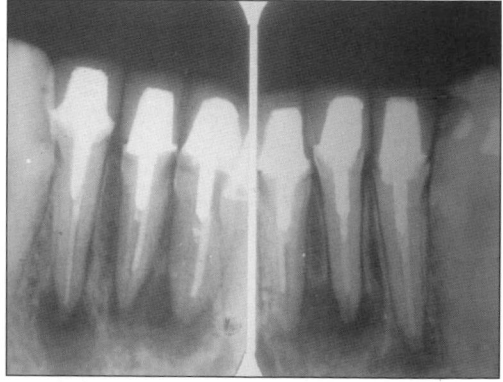

Fig. 2 This case requires complete dismantling and orthograde retreatments. Periradicular surgery is unlikely to be successful.

Fig. 3 The only way that this extruded filling material may be removed is by a surgical approach.

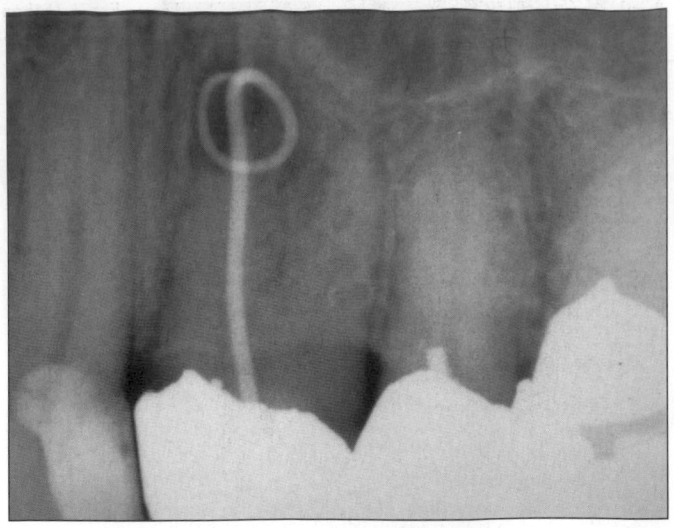

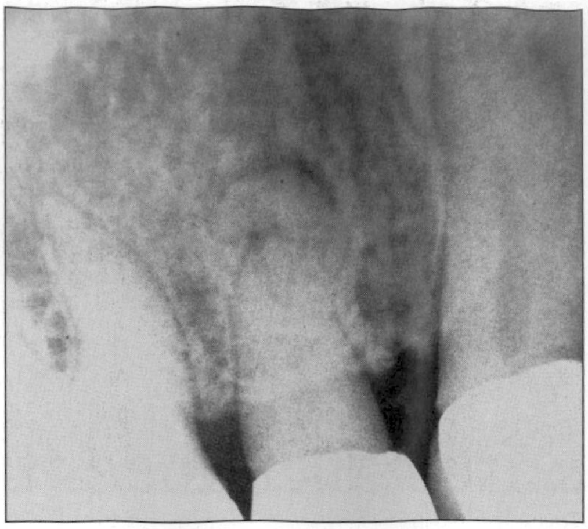

Fig. 4 It would almost certainly be impossible to carry out orthograde root canal treatment on this tooth.

Fig. 5 The pulpal space in this tooth has been obliterated following trauma. Orthograde access proved impossible.

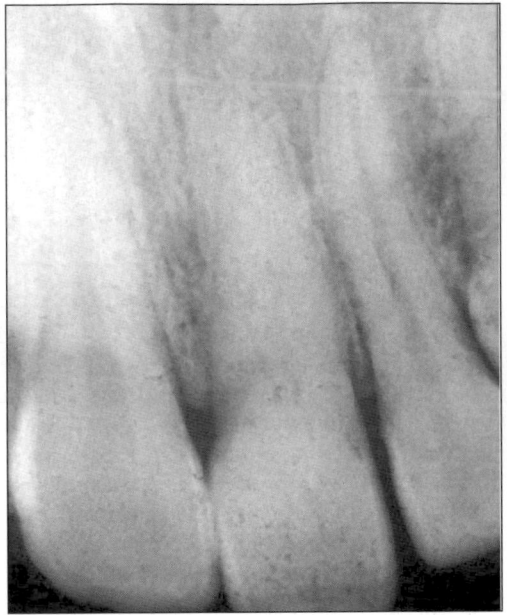

procedures as possible. Alternatively, if these new techniques are not employed, greater consideration should be given to referral for specialist surgical treatment.

INDICATIONS FOR SURGICAL INTERVENTION

Although endodontic surgery is carried out primarily in cases of failed orthograde treatment, there are other indications. Surgery may be necessary to establish drainage, (considered in Part 3); to biopsy a lesion; to repair any defects or perforations in the tooth root; to resect a multirooted tooth where, for technical reasons, one of the roots cannot be successfully treated.

Biopsy of a periapical lesion

The one specific indication for endodontic surgery is uncertainty about the nature of the apical lesion. The lesion should be excised in its entirety and sent for evaluation.

Root-end resection (apicectomy)

The term apicectomy refers to a stage of the operation only. The principal objective is to seal the canal system at the apical foramen from the periradicular tissues. To do this it is necessary to resect the apical part of the root to gain access to the root canal, hence the term. Root-end resection must be an adjunct measure to orthograde root treatment for two reasons. Firstly, there is very little chance of being able to seal all the lateral communications between the canal and the periodontal ligament with a retrograde root-filling technique. Secondly, the area of root-filling material exposed will be greater and the long-term success affected, because all root-filling materials are, to some extent, irritant to the tissues.

Indications for root-end resection

Improvements in root canal treatment techniques have lessened the need for apical surgery. Cases which at first seem obvious candidates for endodontic surgery may respond to conventional treatment provided careful thought is given to the aetiology. Once the decision has been made to carry out surgery, consideration must be given to the chances of success (see Part 12). Access and control of the operating environment are essential, otherwise the end result will be counterproductive.

Retreatment of a failed root filling

Surgery may be considered if a root filling fails and retreatment cannot be effected by orthograde means. There are a number of reasons why a root filling might fail, but generally this is due to inadequate cleansing and filling of the root canal. Some root fillings can prove very difficult to remove, for example hard setting pastes. Occasionally there may be an anatomical reason for the failure, such as an unfilled apical delta. Attempts at retreatment by a conventional orthograde route may be unsuccessful because the original canal cannot be negotiated. Periradicular surgery and root-end filling is therefore justified to ensure that the apical foramen has been sealed.

Root-filling material which has been extruded through the apical foramen may be a contributory cause of failure, since it could be an indication that the apical seal is deficient;

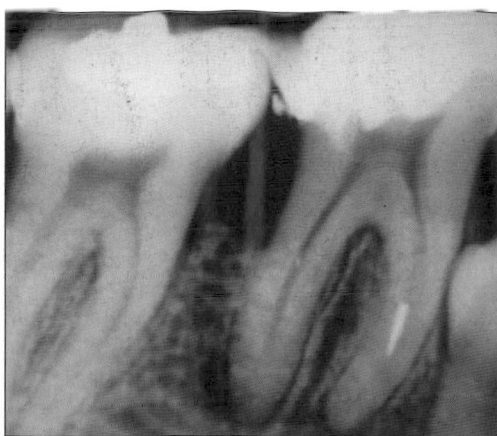

Fig. 6 This fractured instrument in the apical third of the root canal proved impossible to remove.

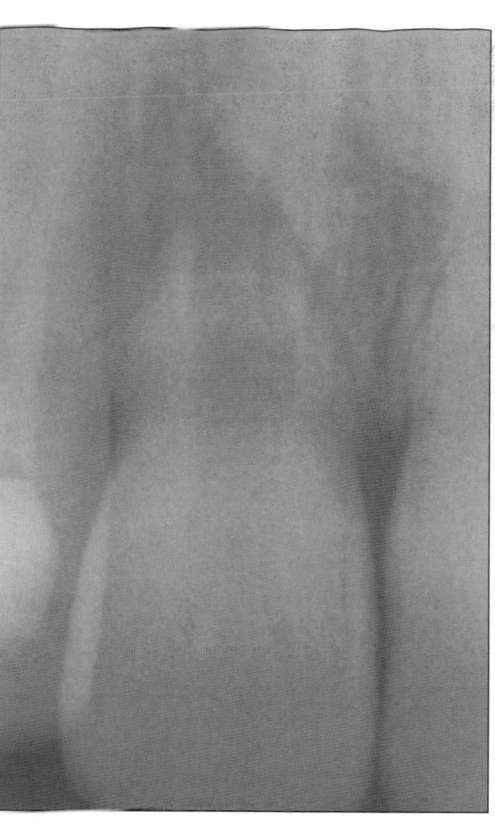

Fig. 7 Orthograde attempts have failed to obturate this tooth with an open apex.

necrotic material may be present at the apex and between the interface of the root filling and the canal wall; the root-filling material itself may be highly irritant (Fig. 3).

PROCEDURAL DIFFICULTIES

During conventional orthograde root canal treatment, problems may arise as a result of one of the following:

- Unusual root canal configurations (Fig. 4).
- Extensive secondary dentine deposition (Fig. 5).
- Fractured instruments within the root canal (Fig. 6).
- Open apex (Fig. 7).
- Existing post in the root canal unfavourable for dismantling (Fig. 8).
- Lateral or accessory canal (Fig. 9).

Unusual root canal configurations

Instrumentation of canals in roots which exhibit bizarre morphology or severe dilaceration may prove impossible. Similarly, where there is an apical delta, thorough cleansing, shaping and obturation of the canal may prove impossible and surgery will be required to complement the orthograde approach.

Extensive secondary dentine deposition

The ageing process results in the deposition of secondary dentine, with a consequent reduction in size of the pulp chamber and the root canal.

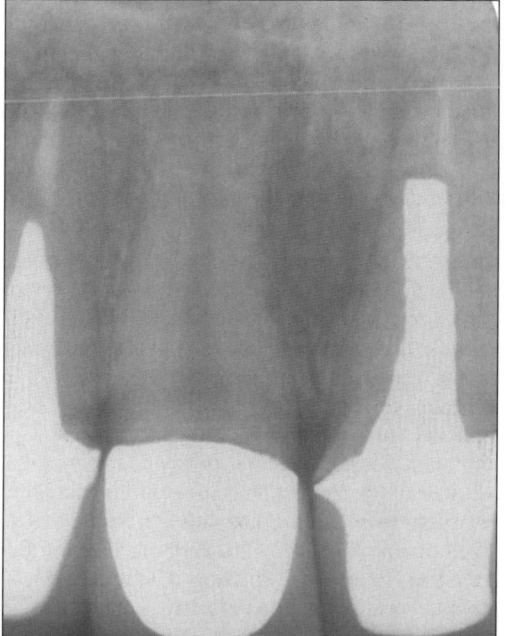

Fig. 8 It was agreed that any attempt to remove the large post and core in tooth 21 (UL1) to permit orthograde retreatment may result in a root fracture. The patient elected for a surgical approach.

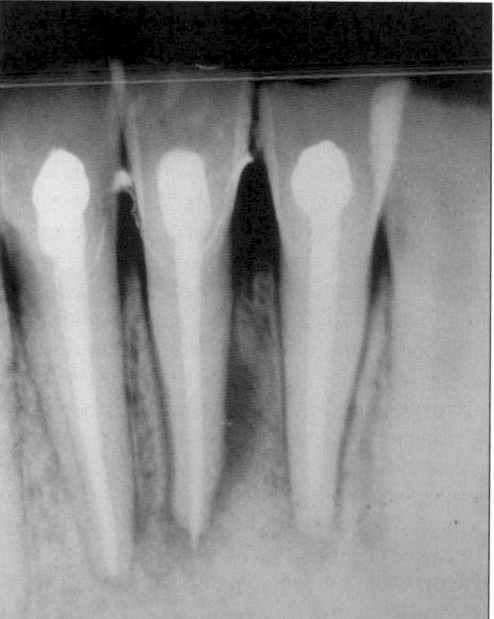

Fig. 9 These lower incisors have been treated but symptoms have persisted at tooth 41 (LR1). The radiograph shows that the periodontitis is centred on the portal of exit from a lateral canal, which still must contain infected debris.

Fig. 10 If this tooth is to be retained with this post perforation, surgical repair will be required.

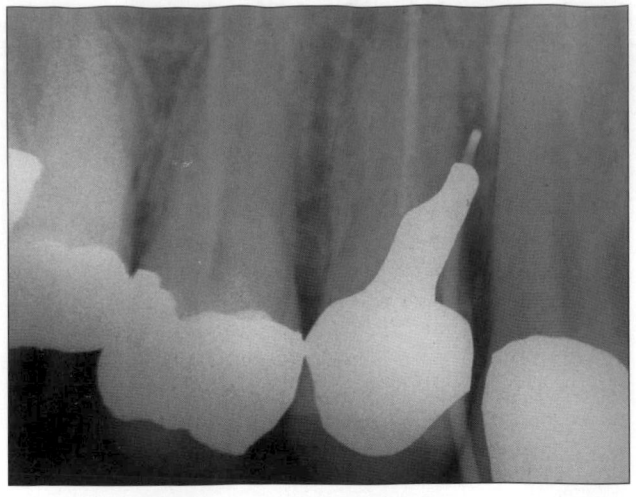

Even more profound sclerosis may result in a tooth which has been subjected to trauma. An asymptomatic irreversible pulpitis may result, bringing about sclerosis of the root canal system. The canals may then be almost completely obliterated and it may prove impossible to identify the canals with even the smallest instruments. Under these circumstances, continued searching deep in the root may result in excessive damage, weakening of the root, or even perforation. Periradicular surgery is then the only alternative to extraction.

Fractured instruments within the root canal

Instruments which have fractured in a root canal do not necessarily result in failure of the root treatment. They should be removed if possible, but if this is impossible, then an attempt should be made to seal the rest of the canal with the instrument in place. Surgery is only necessary if the tooth develops symptoms, or radiographic review shows a failure of healing. The incident should, of course, be recorded in the records, and the patient informed.

Open apex

Teeth that have been injured before root development is complete should be treated conventionally in the first instance. If the pulp is vital, then the coronal pulp is removed and the remaining vital radicular pulp is covered with calcium hydroxide to allow continued root development; this is termed 'apexogenesis'. If the pulp is irreversibly inflamed, then the radicular pulp is removed and the canal filled with calcium hydroxide to encourage root formation and closure of the apex; this is termed 'apexification'.[7]

However, should the treatment fail, then apical surgery may be necessary, to provide an apical seal after completion of the orthograde root filling. Care must be exercised when carrying out this operation as the root structure is often very delicate.

Existing post in the root canal

Periradicular surgery may be indicated for teeth with symptomatic periapical lesions which have satisfactory post crowns in place, provided the root filling in the main body of the canal is satisfactory. However, it has to be remembered that success depends on the canal system being completely sealed. If there is any doubt about this, it is better to remove the crown and post and carry out orthograde root treatment, avoid surgery, and thus provide a sound foundation for any subsequent restoration. Dismantling of post crowns is, however, not always straightforward. An assessment must be made of the length and shape of the post, the strength of the remaining root structure and, if possible, the cement used. Injudicious force during post removal may lead to root fracture and the loss of the tooth. The situation should be discussed in detail with the patient in order that informed consent to the chosen procedure is obtained.[8]

Lateral or accessory canal

Modern endodontic techniques should enable the root canal to be shaped adequately to permit flushing of sodium hypochlorite irrigation throughout the entire root canal system. Unfortunately, infected debris may occasionally persist in lateral or accessory canals. Whilst orthograde retreatment may be attempted, a surgical approach may be the only solution, particularly if these canals form part of the apical delta which may be eliminated by adequate surgical resection.

SURGICAL REPAIR OF ROOTS

Surgery may be necessary to repair defects in a root surface due to either iatrogenic or pathological causes. The two main indications are as follows.

Perforations

Where possible, an orthograde approach should first be used to seal the perforation, ideally using mineral trioxide aggregate (MTA). If this is not practical, the canal must be thoroughly cleaned and filled with calcium hydroxide paste to dry it out and to allow the tissues time to heal. The prepared canal space should then be obturated using conventional root canal filling techniques. Perforations caused by instrumentation errors can usually be treated by an orthograde approach as the access is generally good. However, if clinical symptoms persist or there is bone resorption, or in the case of a large perforation as shown in Figure 10, a surgical approach will be necessary.

Internal and external root resorption

Internal resorption should always be treated by an orthograde route first. If the resorptive process has perforated through to the periodontal ligament, then surgery may be necessary to repair the root and provide an effective seal. Certain types of external root resorption in the early stages can be dealt with by surgery, provided access can be gained to the area (see Root resorption).

Root amputation and hemisection

Periradicular surgery on a posterior tooth is a

more difficult procedure to carry out than on an anterior tooth. For this reason, the relatively simpler techniques of root amputation or hemi-section may be considered. The changes in endodontic and periodontal treatment techniques in recent years have greatly improved the prognosis for this form of treatment. The principal indications are endodontic, restorative or periodontal. Root amputation is an operation where one entire root of a multirooted tooth is removed, leaving the crown intact. Hemisection is the division of a tooth, usually in a buccolingual plane. Normally, one half of the tooth is removed, but both sections may be retained if there is disease in the furcation area only. However, the restorative problems this type of treatment poses are considerable and for this reason the prognosis is generally poor. Pre-operative assessment of both the periodontal and restorative aspects is crucial if these methods of treatment are contemplated.

MEDICAL AND DENTAL CONSIDERATIONS

Although there are few absolute contra-indications to endodontic surgery, a well-documented medical history is essential (see Part 2). In general, heart disease, diabetes, blood dyscrasias, debilitating illnesses and steroid therapy may contra-indicate surgery and special measures are necessary if surgery is contemplated. Consideration must also be given to psychological factors. As a rule, local analgesia is preferable, but patients who are particularly apprehensive may wish to have any surgery carried out under sedation. The choice of anaesthetic may also be governed by the nature of the operation, the site of the tooth and ease of access. A history of rheumatic fever is not a contra-indication for endodontic surgery, provided appropriate antibiotic cover is given. If there is any doubt about a patient's fitness to undergo any surgical endodontic procedure, then the patient's physician should always be consulted.

The first considerations are whether the tooth is worth saving and how important it is in the overall treatment plan. The general state of the mouth should be considered, both hard and soft tissues. The quality of restorative work in the tooth concerned should be particularly noted, and an assessment must also be made of the effects of any proposed surgery on the periodontal condition. The presence of any detectable dehiscence or bony fenestration will influence the design and extent of the flap.

A periapical radiograph should provide all the information required for assessment of the tooth, although it may be necessary to expose more than one film, from different angles. At least 3 mm of the periradicular tissues should be clearly visible. Assessment should be made of the root shape, taking into account any unusual curvature and the number of foramina that may be exposed at the apex as a consequence of the operation. If a sinus is present in the soft tissues, the sinus tract should be visualized by taking a radiograph with a gutta-percha point threaded into the tract, as shown in Part 2, Figure 5.

Good visual access is extremely important, and the anatomy of the area must be thoroughly understood. The position of any major structures such as neurovascular bundles and the maxillary sinus must be noted. A buccal or labial approach is always preferred, as a palatal approach is difficult and should only be undertaken in exceptional circumstances by experienced practitioners.

One of the key factors influencing the success or failure or periradicular surgery is the experience and expertise of the operator. Consideration should always be given to referral to an appropriate specialist, especially in difficult cases. A letter of referral should include a full clinical and medical history, and all relevant radiographs. Both the referring dentist and the specialist providing treatment have a responsibility to obtain informed consent to the procedure.

PERIRADICULAR SURGERY TECHNIQUE

The steps for carrying out this procedure are:

1. Pre-operative care.
2. Anaesthesia and haemostasis.
3. Soft-tissue management.
4. Hard-tissue management.
5. Curettage of area.
6. Resection of root.
7. Retrograde cavity preparation.
8. Retrograde filling.
9. Replacement of flap and suturing.
10. Post-operative care.

Pre-operative care

Although prophylactic antibiotic therapy is not usually required for routine periradicular surgery, systemic antibiotics may be required for any flare-ups prior to surgery. Chlorhexidine mouthwashes may also be beneficial, and these, together with systemic non-steroidal anti-inflammatory drugs, should be considered from the day prior to surgery.[9]

Anaesthesia and haemostasis

Wherever possible, local anaesthesia is the method of choice, although anxious patients who cannot be controlled with tranquillizers may also require intravenous sedation. The local anaesthesia injection also provides haemostasis, essential for good endodontic surgery. Following topical anaesthetic application, an anaesthetic solution with at least 1:80,000 adrenaline is injected slowly into several sites surrounding the surgical field. Local anaesthetic solutions containing Octapressin do not give adequate haemostasis and should be avoided if possible.

In the mandible, block injections should be given, in addition to infiltration of the tissues in the operating area. In the maxilla, the palate must be well infiltrated to anaesthetize the greater palatine nerve. The incisive papilla and canal must also receive sufficient anaesthetic solution to block the long sphenopalatine nerve. The local anaesthetic should be applied at least 10 minutes prior to surgery, to allow profound

Fig. 11 The outline for the incision to raise a) a full muco-periosteal flap, b) a semilunar flap (not recommended), and c) the Luebke-Oschenbein flap.

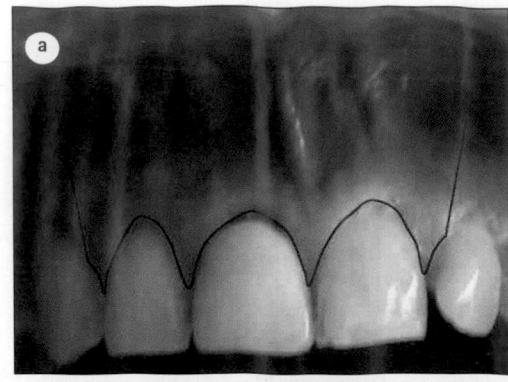

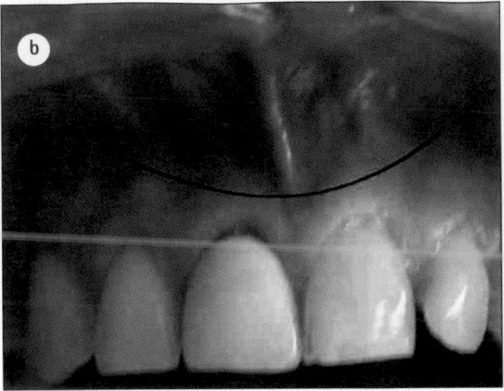

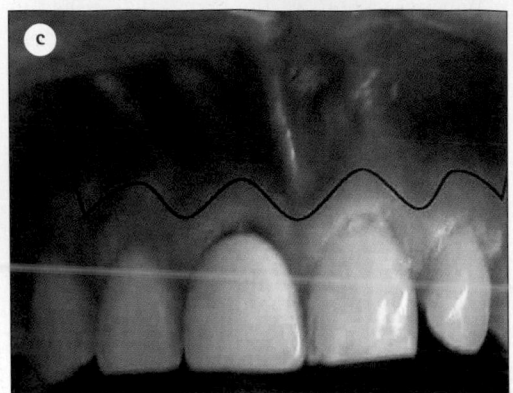

anaesthesia and maximum haemostasis.

Soft-tissue management

The design of the surgical flap should permit an unobstructed view of the operating area and permit easy access for instrumentation. The following points need to be considered:

1. The blood supply to the flap and adjacent tissues must be sufficient to prevent tissue necrosis when it is repositioned.
2. The edges of the flap should lie over sound bone and not cross any void; otherwise breakdown may occur and defective healing will result.
3. Relieving incisions should be vertical, and should not cross any bony eminence, for example the canine eminence, as healing will be poor, particularly if there is a dehiscence or fenestration present.
4. The incision must be clean, so that the flap can be reflected without any tearing of the margins.
5. The flap should always be full thickness and extend to the gingival sulcus. The periodontal tissues should be healthy, as healing will be affected by any overt disease.

There are several designs of flaps, and, whilst the choice may depend upon the size of the lesion, the periodontal status and the state of the coronal tooth structure, it usually depends upon the operator's preference

Full mucoperiosteal flap

This design of flap provides the best possible access to all surgical sites, and can be either a rectangular flap with mesial and distal vertical relieving incisions, or triangular with just one. The former usually provides better access to the

root apex in the anterior part of the mouth, though when operating on posterior teeth the distal relieving incision is not usually necessary, and may prove difficult to suture in the limited space available. The vertical relieving incisions are made firmly down the line angle of the teeth into the gingival crevice, taking in the papilla. The horizontal incision is made along the gingival crevice. The flap is then carefully reflected with a periosteal elevator lifting the periosteum with it from the bone. (Fig. 11a).

Semilunar flap

This flap, where an incision was made in a semi-circle from near the apex of the adjacent tooth, onto the attached gingival, and finishing near the apex of the tooth on the other side, is mentioned purely for historical purposes, and is no longer recommended. Its main disadvantage is the scarring which invariably accompanies this design. However, problems also frequently occurred if the margins of the bony cavity extended across the incision line because the lesion proved to be much larger than was originally apparent (Fig. 11b).

Luebke-Oschenbein flap

The Luebke-Oschenbein flap was designed to overcome some of the disadvantages of the semilunar flap. A vertical incision is made down the distal aspect of the adjacent tooth to a point about 4.0 mm short of the gingival margin. The horizontal incision is scalloped following the contour of the gingival margin through the attached gingivae to the distal aspect of the tooth on the other side. The incision must always be extended to the other side of the fraenum and the distal aspect of the adjacent maxillary central or lateral incisor to avoid a vertical incision next to the fraenum (Fig. 11c).

The flap affords an excellent view of the operating area. However, it still has the disadvantage that the margins of the bony cavity might extend across the incision line, as can happen with the semilunar flap. It is essential to check if there is any periodontal pocketing, as breakdown will then be inevitable. The aim of this flap design is to preserve the integrity of the gingival margins if there are crowns on the teeth. Scarring may again be a problem with this type of flap.

Whatever design is used, the raised flap should be protected from damage during the operation, and should not be allowed to become desiccated.

Hard-tissue management

If the lesion has perforated the cortical plate, then location is a fairly simple matter. However, if this is not the case, then measurement of the tooth from the radiograph taken with a long-cone paralleling technique must be made. Initially, a large size round bur, cooled by copious water or sterile saline, may be used to provide small, shallow exploratory holes to locate the site of the apex and the lesion. This must be done very carefully, to avoid damaging the root surfaces of the teeth in the immediate area. Alternatively, a round bur, again carefully cooled, may be used to locate the apex by paring away the cortical bone over the apex. The bone is shaved away with a very light motion to reduce the heat generated and improve visibility. Sufficient bone should be removed using the bur and curettes until good visual access to the root end is obtained.

Periradicular curettage

The object of this procedure is to remove any soft-tissue lesion with curettes from around the root apex. It may not be possible to remove all the soft tissue until the root end has been resected.

Periradicular curettage used to be a routine operation carried out by many practitioners after completion of a root canal filling. The rationale for this is no longer accepted, because if the root filling has been carried out successfully and the canal system has been sealed, then healing of the lesion will take place without surgical intervention.

When undertaking periradicular surgery, as much as possible of the periapical lesion should be removed. However, the soft tissues in a periapical lesion are essentially reparative and defensive in nature and if other anatomical structures are liable to be damaged some tissue may be left. This is fortunate as, technically, it is difficult to remove every trace of the lesion, especially if it is firmly attached to the wall of the bone cavity.

Pathological material removed should be sent for histopathological examination with full clinical details.

Armamentarium

For all surgical procedures, instruments should

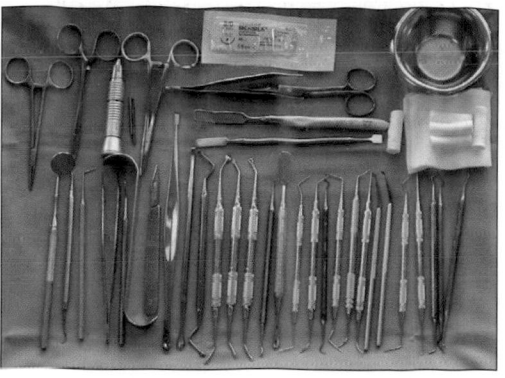

Fig. 12 The sterile instruments necessary for periradicular surgery should be laid out as shown before surgery commences. These include micromirrors and other specialist instruments for performing such surgery using a surgical operating microscope.

be set out, preferably in the order in which they will be used. A typical layout is shown in Figure 12, and includes the modern microsurgical instruments. Magnification, with either optical loupes or a surgical microscope, is preferable.

Resection of the root

The aim of resection is to present the surface of the root so that the apical limit of the canal can be visually examined and to provide access for retrograde cavity preparation. Approximately 3 mm of root is removed which will include almost all lateral canals.[10] It is not necessary to resect the apex to the base of the bony cavity. If too much root is removed, then a greater cross-section of the canal will be revealed, exposing a larger area of filling material to the tissues, and thus reducing the chances of successful healing. The amount of available root length has to be considered for any future post crown construction. There is also an inherent disadvantage as the crown–root ratio is reduced, which may affect the adaptive response of the periodontal ligament to excessive occlusal forces.

A straight fissure bur is used with copious water spray at right angles to the long axis of the tooth. Older textbooks may describe bevelling of the cut root surface at approximately 45° to the long axis of the tooth. This is no longer recommended as this form of resection may result in both incomplete removal of the apical delta, and unnecessary enlargement of the exposed root canal.[11] Magnification is strongly recommended for this procedure, both for accuracy in visualizing the true angulation of the long axis, and also for detailed inspection of the cut root surface and root canal.

Retrograde cavity preparation

Root-end preparation should ideally be performed with a piezo-electric ultrasonic handpiece. If this is not available then a small, round bur should be used in a miniature-headed handpiece, to prepare a single surface cavity to include the entire root canal. Care must be taken to ensure that the canal is penetrated sufficiently far for an effective seal to be placed. Inaccuracy may result in a cavity that is both too large and too shallow. The clinician practising without the aid of magnification must be aware of these difficulties, and the consequent reduction in prognosis of the surgery.

It is now recommended therefore that the ret-

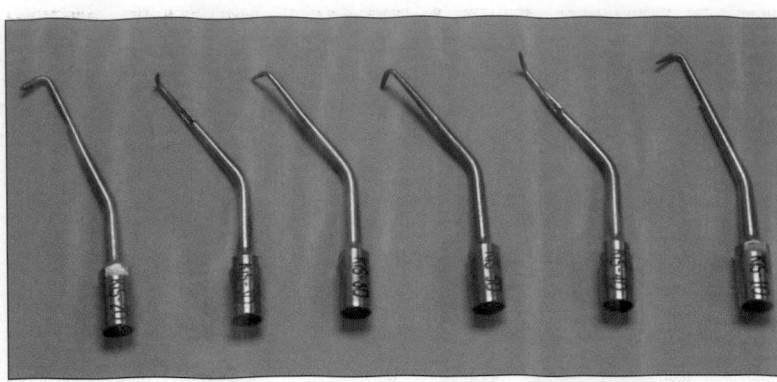

Fig. 13 Ultrasonic KiS® tips for root-end cavity preparation.

rograde cavity is prepared with specially designed ultrasonic tips used in a piezo-electric handpiece. These were first introduced in the early 1990s and the KiS® tips are illustrated in Figure 13.[12] Used with a gentle planing motion along the canal configuration, at a low power setting, a depth of 3 mm may be prepared quickly and cleanly. The cavity should be examined carefully before proceeding to restoration.

Retrograde filling

Before the retrograde filling is inserted, haemostasis must be achieved. Dry epinephrine-impregnated cotton wool balls may be placed into the bony cavity, and will also provide a barrier to prevent accidental loss of excess filling material around the root. Bone wax or ribbon gauze may also be used to isolate the root tip. If gauze is used, it may be wetted with local anaesthetic solution or saline once it is in place, then dabbed dry with a cotton wool pledget. Any excess filling material is more easily retained by the damp gauze.

A biologically compatible material should be used, and amalgam is no longer recommended. A reinforced zinc oxide–eugenol cement such as IRM (modified by the addition of 20% polymethacrylate) or Super EBA (modified with the addition of ethoxybenzoic acid) is recommended. Reinforced glass-ionomer cements or composite resin may be used, although these materials are more technique sensitive.

However, especially when microsurgery is being employed with appropriate magnification, mineral trioxide aggregate (MTA) (Fig. 14) is recommended.[5] It is the least toxic, the most bio-compatible, hydrophilic and gives the best seal. The root end should be dried with paper points or a fine air syringe, and the material may be placed in small increments using a carrier such as the one illustrated in Figure 16a. Alternatively, the MTA may be condensed into a tube shape using the device illustrated in Figure 16b, when it may be carried to the operation site on a probe. Once placed and compacted into the cavity, a damp cotton wool pledget may be used to compress the material and remove excess. Note carefully that the dental surgery assistant must ensure that all instruments, especially the carriers, are thoroughly cleaned of every trace of MTA immediately following surgery, or they may become clogged and rendered useless.

Whichever material is selected for the restoration, it should be thoroughly compacted into the cavity with a small plugger to ensure a dense fill, and burnished with a ball-ended instrument to a smooth finish. The bony cavity should be carefully debrided to ensure that all materials and debris are removed.

Replacement of flap and suturing

Once the retrograde filling has been completed, the packing around the root removed and final debridement carried out, the flap may be sutured into place. Where possible, synthetic monofilament sutures should be used as these do not cause wicking of bacteria into the surgical site and lead to better healing than when silk sutures are used. Resorbable sutures are not recommended.

The vertical relieving incisions should be repaired with interrupted sutures. The gingival margin should be carefully repositioned and

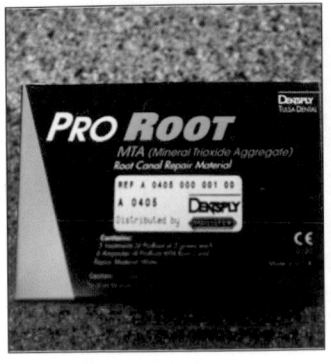

Fig. 14 The commercial presentation of mineral trioxide aggregate

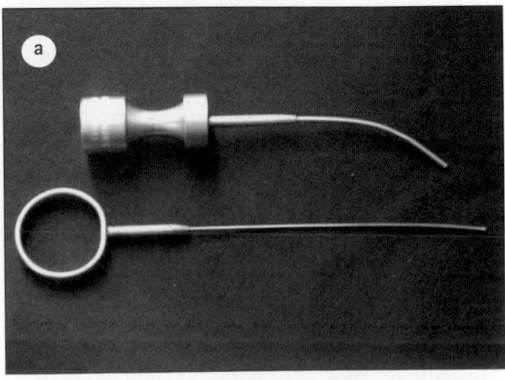

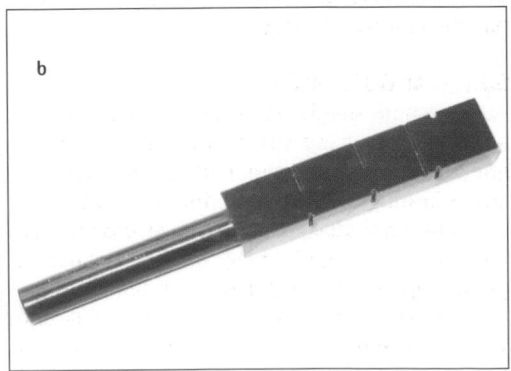

Fig. 15 a) The Dovgan applicator for MTA, available with either a straight or flexible tip. b) A block for compacting and manipulating mixed MTA.

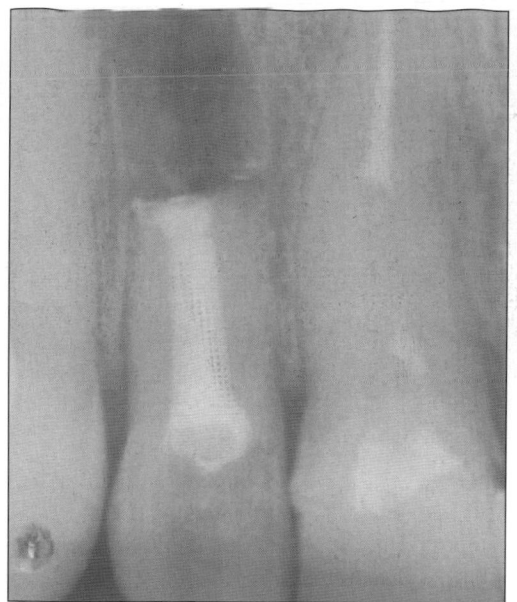

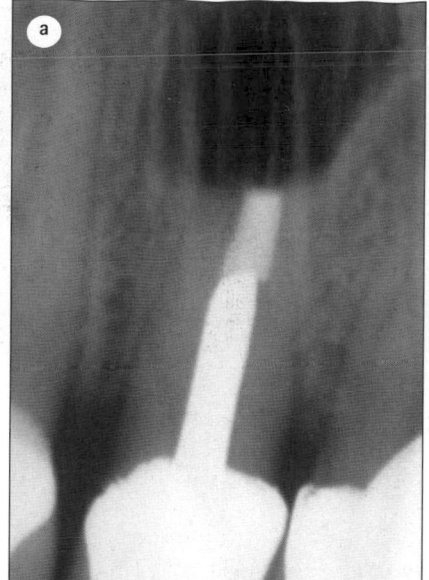

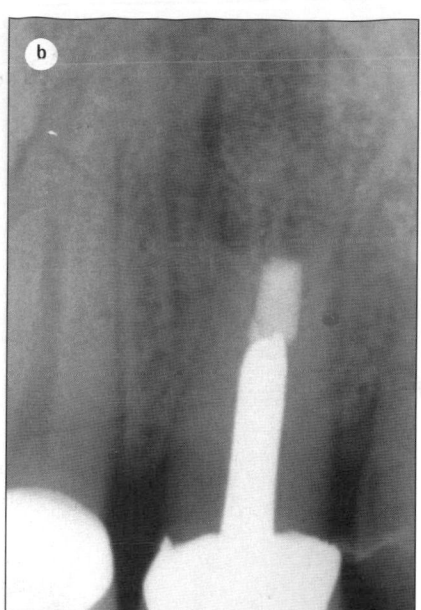

Fig. 16 This tooth has been subject to repeated surgical procedures, without success.

Fig. 17 The radiograph shown at: a) was exposed immediately post-surgery and b) The radiograph taken 1 year later, as part of surgical audit, shows complete healing.

sutured with sling sutures. Commencing at a buccal papilla, the suture is taken through the embrasure, around the tooth and back through the adjacent embrasure to enter the next papilla. The suture is then taken back round the tooth to the original site and the knot tied over the buccal papilla. The sutures may be removed after 48 hours, and certainly no more than 3–4 days, when the periodontal fibres will have reattached. Sutures left longer than this may actually delay healing by wicking.

POST-OPERATIVE CARE

Immediately following suturing, the tissues should be firmly compressed with a damp gauze for 5 minutes. Post-operative swelling can be reduced by the continued application of cold compresses (crushed ice cubes placed in a plastic bag surrounded by a clean soft cloth) for up to 6 hours. Post-operative pain may be controlled by the administration of a long-acting local anaesthetic at the end of the surgery, and by the prescription of non-steroidal anti-inflammatory drugs (NSAIDs). Chlorhexidine mouthwash should be used to keep the surgical site clean until the sutures are removed. The prescription of antibiotics is only necessary if required by the patient's medical history.

SURGICAL OUTCOMES

A radiograph should be exposed either immediately following treatment or when the sutures are removed for comparison with future films to assess healing. Ideally, cementum and periodontal ligament should regenerate over the resected root apex, although in many cases repair occurs by the formation of a fibrous scar. It is reported that success rates may vary between 30% and 80%.[13,14] It should be noted, however, that recent papers have reported treatment using the modern techniques described here to have success rates as high as 92%.[15]

Should failure occur, the cause must be established before further intervention. Repeat surgery has a low success rate, as can be seen in Figure 16. All surgical treatment should, of course, be encompassed within audit and clinical governance, both for the patient and the clinician (Fig. 17).

1   Kim S. Principles of endodontic surgery. *Dent Clin North Am* 1997; **41**: 481–497.
2   Peters L, Wesselink P. Soft tissue management in endodontic surgery. *Dent Clin North Am* 1997; **41**: 513–528.
3   Chindia M L, Valderhaug J. Periodontal status following trapezoidal and semilunar flaps in apicectomy. *East African Med J* 1995; **72**: 564–567.
4   Morgan L A, Marshall J G. A scanning electron microscopic study of in vivo ultrasonic root-end preparations. *J Endod* 1999; **25**: 567–570.
5   Torabinejad M, Pitt Ford T R, Abedi H R, Kariyawasam S P, Tang H M. Tissue reaction to implanted root-end filling materials in the tibia and mandible of guinea pigs. *J Endod* 1998; **24**: 468–471.
6   Kim S. Endodontic Microsurgery. Chapter 19 in Cohen S and Burns RC, *Pathways of the Pulp*. St Louis: Mosby 2002.
7   Webber R T. Apexogenesis versus apexification. *Dent Clin North Am* 1984; **28**: 669–697.
8   Layton S, Korsen J. Informed consent in oral and maxillofacial surgery: a study of the value of written warnings. *Br J Oral Maxillofac Surg* 1994; **32**: 34–36.
9   Martin M V, Nind D. Use of chlorhexidine gluconate for pre-operative disinfection of apicectomy sites. *Br Dent J* 1987; **162**: 459–461.
10 Hsu Y Y, Kim S. The resected root surface. The issue of canal isthmuses. *Dent Clin North Am* 1997; **41**: 529–540.
11 Gilheany P A, Figdor D, Tyas M J. Apical dentin permeability and microleakage associated with root end resection and retrograde filling. *J Endod* 1994; **20**: 22–26.
12 Carr G. Common errors in periradicular surgery. *Endod Rep* 1993; **8**: 12–16.
13 Jansson L, Sandstedt P, Laftman A C, Skogland A. Relationship between apical and marginal healing in periradicular surgery. *Oral Surg, Oral Med, Oral Path, Oral Rad, Endod* 1997; **83**: 596–601.
14 Rud J, Andreasen J O, Jensen J E. Radiographic criteria for the assessment of healing after endodontic surgery. *Int J Oral Surg* 1972; **1**: 195–214.
15 Maddalone M, Gagliani M. Periapical endodontic surgery: a 3-year follow-up study. *Int Endod J* 2003; **36**: 193–198.

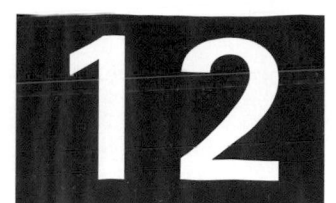

IN BRIEF
- Most problems in root canal treatment could have been avoided with care and attention to treatment principles. Careful examination of the pre-operative radiograph is essential.
- It is possible to remove most fractured instruments, posts and failed root filings if the correct aids are to hand, and magnification is available.
- It is essential that practitioners know the prognosis for different endodontic procedures, both from the endodontic literature and their own clinical experience.

Endodontic problems

If modern clinical techniques were carefully followed, many common endodontic problems would never occur. Incorrectly designed access cavities may make root canals both difficult to identify and to instrument. Careful study of the pre-operative radiograph is essential. Various aids are available to remove fractured instruments and failed root fillings, but the problem must first be correctly diagnosed. As more patients seek cosmetic procedures, the practitioner should be familiar with the 'walking bleach' procedure, again after careful diagnosis of the cause of the discolouration. The practitioner should also be fully aware of the prognosis for this and other endodontic procedures.

Endodontics is a skill requiring the use of delicate instruments in confined spaces. Inevitably, problems will occur, but many of these are avoidable providing the operator exercises care and patience. A few tips on how to overcome some of these problems will be given in this part. Should the reader require a more wide-ranging and detailed account, specialist endodontic textbooks on this subject may be referred to.[1]

ACCESS

It is important to have good visual access and sufficient space to allow direct line access into the apical third of the root canal. A useful way of assessing a patient for molar endodontics is that the operator should be able to place two fingers between the maxillary and mandibular incisors. If this is not possible owing to a small mouth or limited opening, then it may be unwise to commence root canal therapy. Assessing access for posterior surgical endodontics may be done by retracting the lip at the corner of the mouth with a finger; the surgical area should be directly visible.

The general guidelines for access cavities have already been discussed in Part 6. However, there are occasions when these should be adapted to suit a particular case. Inadequate access will lead to poor treatment and, unless the endodontic treatment is successful, further restoration of the tooth is irrelevant.

Before cutting the access cavity, the extent and type of final restoration should be borne in mind. If an anterior tooth will require a crown following the root treatment, the access cavity could be cut on the labial surface (Fig. 1). In posterior teeth it may be advantageous to reduce the walls, if either they are already weakened or there is a crown or root fracture.

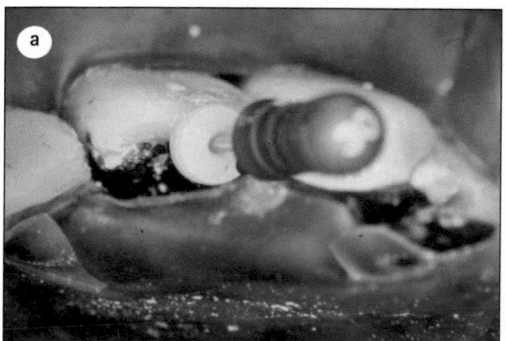
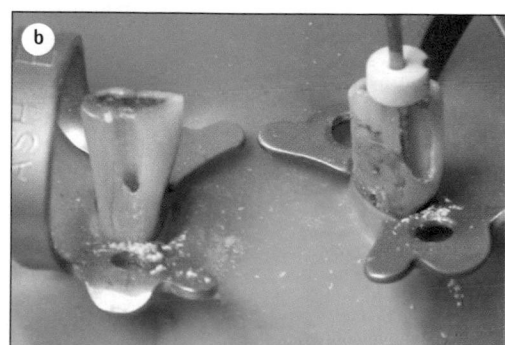

Fig. 1 Unconventional access cavities may be used in some situations. a) A resin-retained bridge had been fitted to replace UL1 (21) lost through trauma. When a periapical lesion developed related to UR1 (11), an access cavity was cut through the incisal edge. b) The last standing teeth are to be cut down for overdenture abutment.

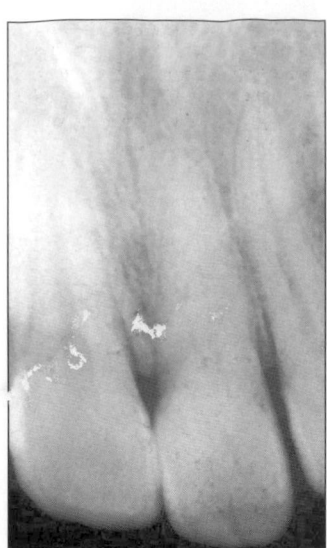

Fig. 2 A radiograph of tooth UL1 (21), which suffered trauma 5 years previously, showing no apparent sign of a root canal system.

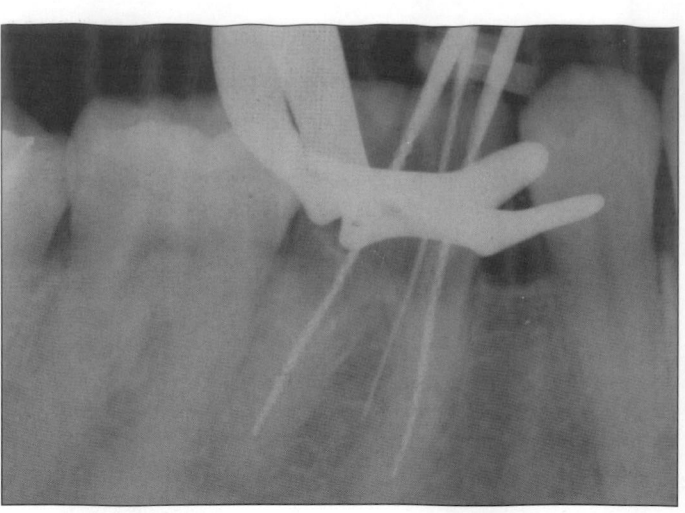

Fig. 3 The operator was unable to locate the access to the mesiobuccal canal. A small, round bur was used to explore the area, and an orifice was found. Unfortunately a radiograph revealed that a perforation into the furcation had been created. As the pulp chamber was clean and well isolated, the perforation was repaired with resin-modified glass-ionomer cement and the tooth remained symptomless.

LOCATING AND NEGOTIATING FINE CANALS

Many root canals, particularly in the elderly patient, are difficult to locate. The pulp chambers may be sclerosed or contain large pulp stones and the root canals may be so fine that even when located they are difficult to negotiate.

Dentine deposition occurs as a response to any moderate injury to the pulp, in particular luxation injuries. Initially, the pulp chamber reduces in size, followed by a gradual narrowing of the root canals. The incidence of pulpal necrosis following canal obliteration is not high and so does not warrant intervention by elective root canal treatment.[2]

Radiographs of teeth showing apparent total canal obliteration are deceptive (Fig. 2). Cvek *et al.* report a study in which attempts were made to locate and negotiate root canals which were not visible on the pre-operative radiographs.[3] In 54 incisors with periapical lesions, the root canal was located and treated in all but one of them.

These narrow canals may take time to locate. The pre-operative radiograph contains useful information: the size, curvature and position of the root canal(s) in relation to the pulp chamber may be noted. A meticulous search must be made of the floor of the pulp chamber with either an endodontic (DG16) probe or an 08 or 10 file. The floor of the pulp chamber is darker than the walls and the canal entrances are situated, in posterior teeth, at each corner. Fibre-optic light, transilluminating the tooth, and magnification using either binocular loupes or an operating microscope as discussed in Part 4 are also of assistance.

If the canal cannot be located, an ultrasonic tip as described in Part 5 may be used to break down secondary dentine from the floor of the pulp chamber around the anticipated canal opening. As a final resort it will be necessary to drill using a small, round bur in a slow running standard handpiece. A bur hole, approximately 2.00 mm in depth, is then drilled at the expected site of the canal along the main axis of the root. A radiograph is taken with the bur *in situ* and the direction of the bur corrected if further drilling is necessary. This can be a frustrating exercise and numerous fine files will be

damaged as the tips curve in the round shape produced by the bur. The associated risks of perforation do mean that this really is a 'last resort', as shown in Figure 3.

Once the entrance has been located, the next step is to negotiate the canal using a fine instrument. A curve is placed at the tip of an 06 or 08 hand file. It is useful to dip the tip of the instrument into a lubricant such as Hibiscrub. The instrument is gradually advanced into the canal using a small, contrarotating, 'watchwinding' movement to advance the file. Force should not be used. The curve in the instrument tip will seek the path of least resistance and allow the instrument to penetrate further into the canal. A push–pull filing motion may then be used to free coronal obstructions in the canal. The file is removed, copious irrigation used and the procedure repeated until the canal is negotiated to the working length. If an electronic apex locator is not being used it will be necessary to enlarge the canal with successively larger fine instruments up to a size 15 before confirming the working length, as an 06 file may not be seen accurately on a diagnostic radiograph.

EDTA paste (ethylenediamine tetra-acetic acid) is not recommended for the initial negotiation of the canal, as it is a chelating agent. The walls of the dentine will be softened, which means a false canal could be cut. EDTA paste is, however, extremely useful when preparing the canal walls once the full length has been negotiated.

LEDGED OR BLOCKED CANALS

Incorrect technique in preparation can lead to either obstruction of the root canal with pulpal debris, compacted dentine and other debris, or the formation of a ledge in the wall of the canal.

In the case of a ledged canal (Fig. 4), a curve should be placed near the tip of a fine hand instrument, the canal irrigated with sodium hypochlorite, and the instrument inserted into the canal. The notch in the rubber stop should be aligned with the curve so that the instrument tip may be directed away from the ledge and gradually advanced with small contrarotating movements. Once the instrument is beyond the ledge a short push–pull filing motion is used to reduce the ledge in the curve before removing the file. A lubricant such as EDTA paste is useful to help remove the ledge. This is not a difficult procedure once the ledge has been bypassed. A canal that has been blocked with pulpal or dentine debris may well be impossible to negotiate. Copious irrigation, the use of EDTA paste and a very fine instrument may be tried. The danger is of either packing the debris harder into the canal or creating a false canal.

RE-ROOT TREATMENT

A root filling may have to be removed and the tooth retreated for a variety of reasons. The patient may be experiencing symptoms, a periapical radiolucency may be increasing in size, or the coronal restoration may require replacing in a tooth where the root filling is inadequate. Whatever the reason, the first step is to identify the type of filling material that has been used (Fig. 5) and to assess the difficulty of the procedure. The method used to remove the previous root filling will depend on the type of material used.

Paste

A soft root-filling material may be removed easily with Hedstroem files and copious irrigation.

Cement

Some cements set hard and have apparently no solvent and, as a result, are almost impossible to remove. The first stage in attempting to remove a cement is to flood the canal entrance with chloroform or xylene and use an endodontic probe and then Hedstroem files. If this fails, the coronal 2–3 mm can be removed with a small rosehead bur followed by files. Alternatively, ultrasonics may be used to break down the cement and flush out the debris. It may, however, prove impossible to negotiate a canal filled with a hard setting cement.

Gutta-percha

Gutta-percha is simple to remove. Gates–Glidden burs may be used first to gain access to the root canal. The burs both cut away gutta-percha, and soften it by the frictional heat of rotation. There are various solvents for gutta-percha, which may be dispensed into a Dappens dish and picked up on the tip each instrument. Chloroform, halothane and xylene may be available in the surgery, or oil of eucalyptus and oil of turpentine are both effective. Once access has been made it is usually possible to remove the remainder of the gutta-percha with conventional filing techniques.

Alternatively, nickel-titanium rotary instruments are very efficient for softening and removing gutta-percha from canals that will accommodate them. Initial exploration with hand files is necessary to create room for the cutting flutes of the instruments. They should not be used to path-find. The piezo-electric ultrasonic machines are also useful as their heat generation aids removal of softened gutta-percha. Specially designed tips are available for this procedure.

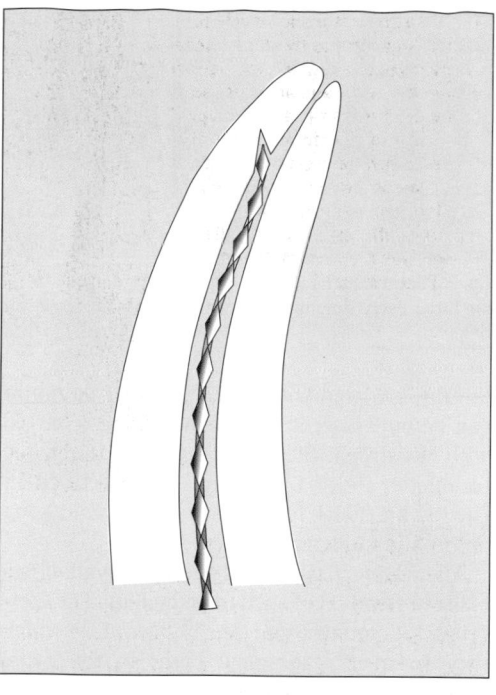

Fig. 4 A diagram of a canal with a ledge in the outer curve, showing how the tip of a pre-curved file may enter the ledge. If the file is rotated through 180° the curved tip will follow the original canal.

If the original gutta-percha filling has been extended beyond the apical foramen, removal may prove impossible. One method proposed for this situation involves first creating a gap between the material and the wall of the canal with a canal probe. A Hedstroem file may then be carefully 'screwed' into the space. A second and, if possible, third file are similarly inserted into the mass of the gutta-percha. The handles of the files are grasped, and a steady withdrawal force exerted to remove the gutta-percha point(s). Hedstroem files are needed to grip and pull back the gutta-percha.

Metal points

The method of removing silver or titanium points is dictated by their position within the root canal. Silver points are easier to remove if there has been leakage of tissue fluids into the canal and corrosion has occurred.

The simplest situation is when the coronal end of the point protrudes far enough into the pulp chamber so that it may be grasped by either Steiglitz forceps (Fig. 6), narrow-beaked artery forceps or fine pliers.

If the point lies in the root canal below the pulp chamber but in a straight part of the canal, attempts should be made to bypass and either remove the point or incorporate it into the root filling. A size 08 or 10 file or reamer is used, and

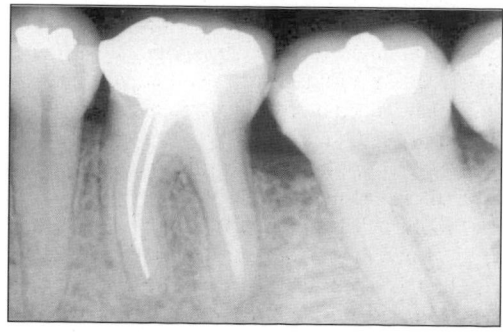

Fig. 5 This tooth has been root filled using both silver points and gutta-percha. The operator must be able to distinguish between various root-filling materials by their radiographic appearance.

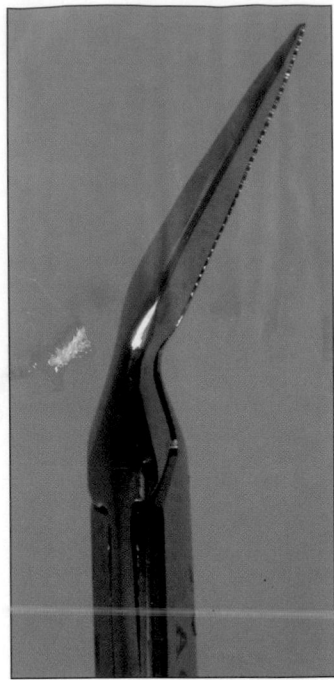

Fig. 6 Steiglitz forceps have long narrow beaks, and are useful for grasping broken instruments in the pulp chamber.

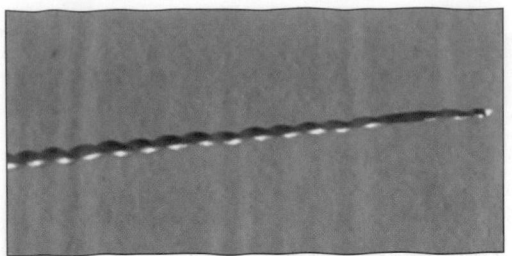

Fig. 7 Files should be visually inspected for damage to the flutes every time they are removed from the tooth for cleaning.

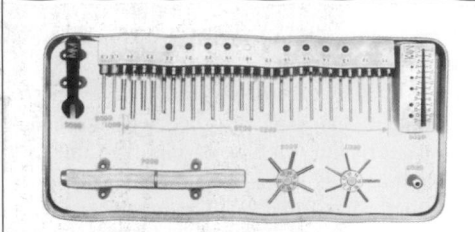

Fig. 8 A Masserann kit for removal of fractured instruments and posts.

the tip is coated with EDTA paste. If the point can be bypassed, it can frequently be removed with Hedstroem files or by using an ultrasonic technique. CPR® Ultrasonic tips (described in Part 5) are ideal for accessing and dislodging points and broken instruments.

Alternatively, two fine devices are available to assist in removal of such impediments. The Cancellier kit contains four fine hollow tubes which may fit over a loosened point in the canal enabling its withdrawal. The Meitrac Endo Safety System involves the use of a mini-trephine to free the tip of the fractured point. This may then be gripped using two 'locking' tubes and withdrawn.

Unless an operating microscope is used, it is seldom possible to remove a point which is lodged in the apical third of a curved root canal. Attempts should be made either to bypass the fragment and incorporate it into the root filling, or condense gutta-percha vertically up to the obstruction, with a view to apical surgery should signs of failure occur.

FRACTURED INSTRUMENTS

The time required to remove or bypass a fractured instrument from the root canal far outweighs the simple precautions that should be taken routinely to prevent such an occurrence. The simple rules which will prevent instrument fracture are as follows.

1. Each time an endodontic instrument is picked up it should be visually checked for any damage or deformation of the twisted flutes (Fig. 7). The assistance of a well-trained dental nurse can be invaluable. Damaged instruments should be discarded immediately.
2. Never force an instrument in the canal.
3. Do not miss out sizes. Although appearing small, moving from a size 10 to a size 15 file

involves an increase in tip diameter of 50%. It is preferable to repeat the use of the smaller file than apply excess force to the next size.
4. When using the balanced force technique, limit rotations to 60° as described by Roane *et al.* and never rotate an instrument more than one quarter turn in a clockwise direction.[4]

The techniques used for removal of a fractured instrument are similar to those described previously for metal points. In addition, the Masserann was specifically designed to extract metal fragments from root canals. The Masserann kit (Fig. 8) consists of a number of trepans with a range of diameters from 1.1 mm to 2.4 mm. The trepans are hollow tubes designed to cut a trough around the metal fragment (Fig. 9). Note that the trepans are designed to be used with an anti-clockwise rotation. This will assist with the removal of any threaded materials which will have a conventional thread. The operator should be particularly aware of this as a potential problem if attempting to remove a fractured Hand File of Greater Taper, which have a reverse thread.

The trough usually has to be cut along at least half the length of the fragment before it is sufficiently loosened to allow its extraction. It is recommended that the trepan is operated by hand, using the special handle provided, and not placed in a handpiece. A feeler gauge from the kit is used to judge the size of the trepan required. EDTA paste will help to lubricate and soften the dentine. The kit also contains a Masserann extractor, which is placed over the end of the loosened fragment so that it may be gripped and removed. If the fragment is too large for the extractor, then a size smaller trepan may be forced over the end of the fragment,

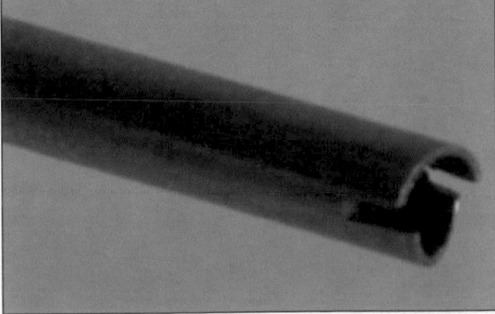

Fig. 9 The tip of the Masserann trepan showing the cutting flutes, designed to cut in an anticlockwise direction.

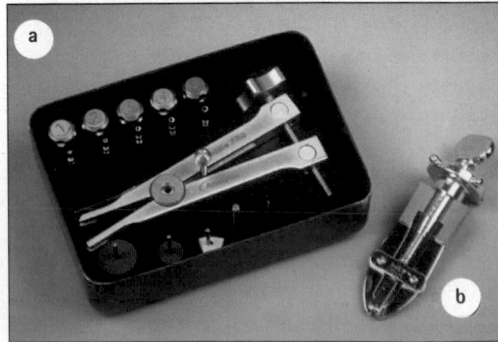

Fig. 10 Post extractors for dismantling post–crowns: a) the Eggler, and b) the Ruddle systems.

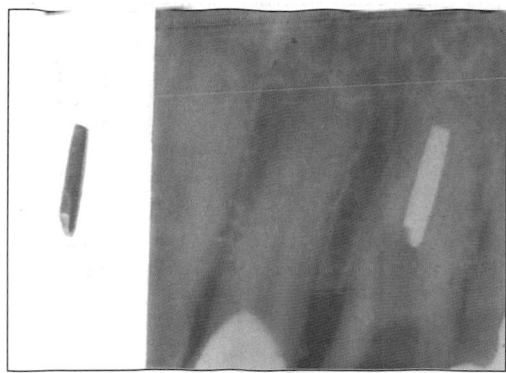

Fig. 11 A fractured post successfully removed with the Masseran kit.

which is then gripped firmly enough to allow its withdrawal from the canal. However, the operator must weigh the benefits of this procedure against the damage to the trepan.

A fractured instrument remaining in a canal does not mean that the attempt at root treatment will fail. It has been demonstrated that, provided the remainder of the root canal is filled conventionally, the success rate is not significantly affected.[5,6]

POSTS

A post may have to be removed because either the tooth requires (re)root filling or the post has fractured. The procedure presents problems as there is a danger of fracturing or perforating the root of the tooth. Threaded posts which have fractured can be removed by cutting a groove in the post end and unscrewing. It is possible to extract a smooth-sided post and core using a post extractor (Fig. 10).

A piezo-electric ultrasonic system, used with special tips, should first be used at the appropriate power setting. Moving the tips around the base of the post at moderate power will remove cement around the post. A different tip may then be used to apply maximum vibratory energy to the post in an attempt to vibrate the post loose directly.

With the Eggler system, the core must first be shaped so that its sides are parallel and capable of being gripped. The mesial and distal shoulders of the crown preparation must be cut to the same

height so there is no torsional force. The post extractor is then placed over the post and the screw tightened onto the core; the feet are then lowered on to the shoulders of the preparation by turning the end knob. Several more turns will ease the post out of the post hole.

With the Ruddle system, a trephine is used to produce a parallel side in the post, which is then grasped in a matching sized thread cutting tap to a maximum depth of 3 mm. The post removal pliers are placed over a rubber cushion, and gently tightened. If removal is difficult, further ultrasonic energy may be applied. As with all such instruments, there is a danger of root fracture, and expertise should be gained in a technical laboratory before attempting these techniques in a clinical situation.

A fractured post lying within the root canal may either be drilled out using a high-speed handpiece, which is a hazardous procedure, or removed with a Masserann kit as described earlier. Figure 11 shows the initial radiograph of the fractured post, and the item successfully removed with the Masseran kit.

VERTICAL ROOT FRACTURE

Although infrequent, this problem may be difficult to diagnose. The patient may present with mild symptoms, or it may appear that the root canal treatment has not been successful. Cases have been reported where the first indication of a vertical root fracture has been when a mucoperiosteal flap has been raised to carry out periradicular surgery on an apparently persistent lesion. Figure 12 in Part 2 shows a tooth with such a fracture which had to be extracted.

The diagnosis can, however, be suspected when a radiograph shows bone loss extending all around a root or a tooth, as in Figure 12. The vertical defect has led to bacterial contamination of the entire tooth surface.

THE DISCOLORED ROOT-FILLED TOOTH

Bleaching and tooth-whitening procedures are rapidly becoming a part of every dentist's practice. The routine use of such materials in restorative dentistry is outside the scope of this text, and the subject is comprehensively cov-

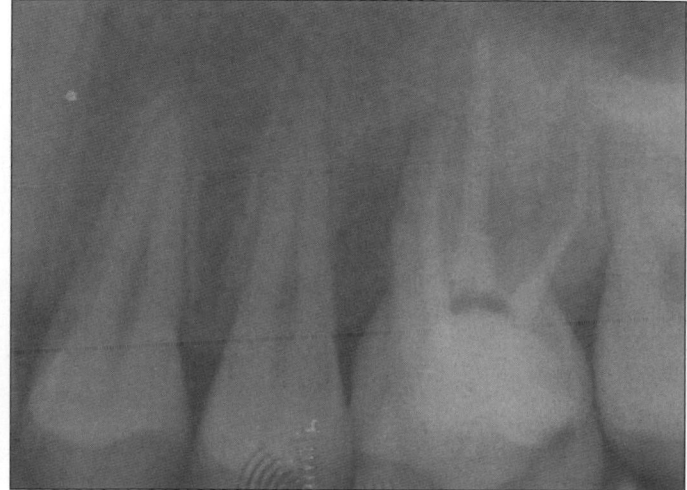

Fig. 12 A radiograph of a molar with a vertical root fracture, showing the pathognomonic appearance of periodontitis surrounding the entire root.

Fig. 13 Internal bleaching has been used to lighten this root canal treated central incisor. Figure courtesy of Dr M Elkhazindar, Glasgow Dental Hospital.

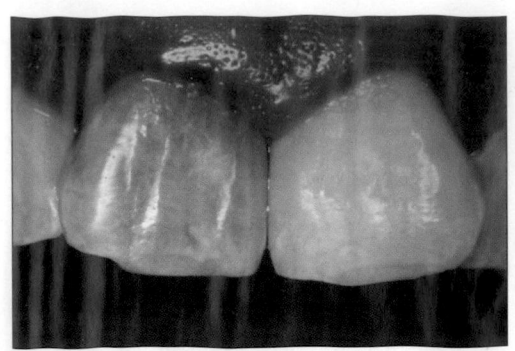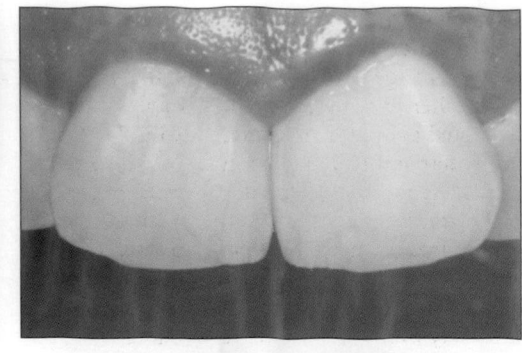

Table 1 Overview of success in endodontic treatment (From Friedman[12])

Treatment procedure	Weighted average success of reports in approximately the past 50 years	Weighted average success of reports in approximately the past 10 years
Endodontic treatment of teeth without periapical periodontitis	34 studies Range from 100% to 67% Weighted average 91%	6 studies Range from 100% to 88% Weighted average 93%
Endodontic treatment of teeth with periapical periodontitis	38 studies Range from 96% to 38% Weighted average 76%	8 studies Range from 94% to 46% Weighted average 77%
Endodontic treatment of teeth with periapical periodontitis using calcium hydroxide intervisit dressing		6 studies since 1987 Range from 86% to 69% Weighted average 79%
Orthograde endodontic retreatment in teeth with periapical periodontitis	9 studies Range from 88% to 48% Weighted average 70%	3 studies Range from 74% to 56% Weighted average 62%
Periradicular surgery in teeth with periapical periodontitis	29 studies Range from 95% to 30% Weighted average 59%	11 studies Range from 81% to 30% Weighted average 63%

ered in other books.[7,8] However, teeth which have been root filled may darken for various reasons, and may benefit from internal bleaching using the technique known as 'walking bleach'. An illustration of the potential can be seen in Figure 13.

It is essential wherever possible to identify the cause of the discoloration. Some of those specifically due to endodontics may be:[9]

- Internal haemorrhage within the dentine following trauma;
- Seepage of toxins from the infected pulpal contents;
- Staining from medicaments, cements, etc., particularly those containing silver;
- The optical effects of dehydration.

Briefly, the normally recommended technique is as follows:

1. Clean and polish all the teeth thoroughly to remove any extrinsic stain.
2. Match the existing shade of the tooth with a ceramic shade guide (if possible with an intra-oral photograph of the tooth and tab).
3. Isolate the tooth with rubber dam, sealing the margins carefully around the teeth with a caulking agent.

4. Remove the restoration from the access cavity, ensuring that all aspects are clean.
5. Clean out all endodontic materials from the pulp chamber, to a depth of 2 mm into the root canal.
6. Seal the root filling with a layer of glass-ionomer cement of the lightest shade.
7. Soak a cotton pledget in 30% hydrogen peroxide and place in the access cavity.
8. Apply a heated instrument to the pledget, and repeat the process several times. (Note that in a recent comprehensive review of this procedure Attin *et al.* suggest that the use of 30% hydrogen peroxide and the application of heat may both contribute to the initiation of cervical resorption.[10])
9. Place a mixture of sodium perborate and 3% hydrogen peroxide in the pulp chamber, and seal it in place with a non-eugenol temporary cement. This constitutes the 'walking-bleach' phase of the procedure.
10. Review the patient after one week, and measure the change in colour.
11. The procedure may require repeating several times.
12. The access cavity should be restored completely with the lightest paediatric shade of composite resin.

PROGNOSIS IN ENDODONTICS

All endodontic procedures should be reviewed as part of audit and clinical governance. An assessment of the degree of healing or otherwise must be made, and unsatisfactory results may require either further monitoring or retreatment. However, it should be noted that Ørstavik reported that over 75% of apical periodontitis lesions developing after endodontic treatment can be observed radiographically after one year.[11] It may be considered therefore that if healing is evident after one year, further radiographic monitoring is not indicated.

One method of monitoring would be to employ the Periapical Index (PAI) described by Ørstavik *at al.*[12] Standard radiographic views are presented of five apical conditions, and the operator compares their own result with these standards. A score of 1 indicates normal periapical appearance; 2 indicates slight disorganization of the bone texture; 3 loss of bone and unusual bone pattern; 4 shows classic periapical periodontitis; and 5 is similar, but with obvious wider spread.

Many studies have been reported on the success of endodontic treatment, many assessing the result against the PAI. Friedman reports a comprehensive review of these studies, and the weighted averages are summarized in Table 1.[13] Particular note should be made of the significantly reduced weighted average prognosis when treating teeth presenting with an established area of periapical periodontitis seen on radiographic examination. These figures should be studied by the clinician, and an estimate of the likely prognosis should form part of the procedure of obtaining informed or valid consent.

1. Guttman, J L, Dumsha T C, Lovdahl P E, Hovland E J. *Problem Solving in Endodontics.* 3rd Ed. St Louis: Mosby, 1997.

2. Andreasen J O, Andreasen F M. Chapter 9 in *Textbook and colour atlas of traumatic injuries to the teeth.* 3rd Ed. Denmark: Munksgard, 1994.

3. Cvek M, Granath L-E, Lundberg M. Failures and healing in endodontically treated non-vital anterior teeth with post-traumatically reduced pulpal lumen. *Acta Odont Scand* 1982; **40**: 223–228.

4. Roane J B, Sabala C L, Duncanson M G. The balanced force concept for instrumentation of curved canals. *J Endod* 1985; **11**: 203–211

5. Crump M C, Natkin E. Relationship of broken root canal instruments to endodontic case prognosis: a clinical investigation. *J Am Dent Assoc* 1970; **80**: 1341–1347.

6. Lumley P J. Management of silver points and fractured instruments. *CPD Dentistry* 2000; **1**: 87–92.

7. Greenwall L. *Bleaching techniques in restorative dentistry.* London: Martin Dunitz, 2001.

8. Sheets C G, Paquette, J M, Wright R S. Chapter 21 in Cohen S & Burns R C. *Pathways of the Pulp,* Eighth Ed. St Louis: Mosby, 2002.

9. Nathoo S A. The chemistry and mechanisms of extrinsic and intrinsic discoloration. *J Am Dent Assoc* 1997; **128**: 6S–10S.

10. Attin T, Paqué F, Ajam F, Lennon Á. Review of the current status of tooth whitening with the walking bleach technique. *Int End J* 2003; **36**: 313–329.

11. Ørstavik D. Time-course and risk analyses of the development and healing of chronic apical periodontitis in man. *Int Endod J* 1996; **29**: 150–155

12. Ørstavik D, Kerekes K and Eriksen H M. The periapical index: A scoring system for radiographic assessment of periapical periodontitis. *Endod Dent Traumatol* 18; 2: 20–34.

13. Friedman S. Treatment outcome and prognosis of endodontic therapy. In Ørstavik D, Pitt Ford T R, *Essential Endodontology.* Oxford: Blackwell Science, 1998

Index

ENDODONTICS